DYSLEXIA MY LIFE

One man's story of his life with
a learning disability.

AN

AUTOBIOGRAPHY

Anne :) thanks 4 helping so many !!

By *GIRARD J. SAGMILLER*
With *Gigi Lane*

Library Of Congress #95-083487
ISBN 0-9643087-1-1

CONTENTS

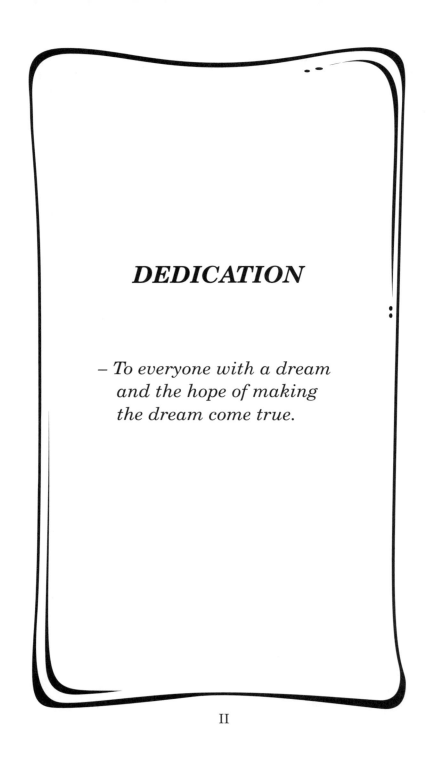

DEDICATION

*– To everyone with a dream
and the hope of making
the dream come true.*

ACKNOWLEDGMENTS

I would like to thank Valerie Russell and Marilyn Ray for editing this book, Gigi Lane for helping, and Michael Hage for taking the photos. Most of all, I want to thank all the people that stood beside me, not in front or behind but beside me, to help reach my goals in life. Last, I thank you for buying the book—may it fuel your learning and goal desires.

INTRODUCTION

This is the story of my life as a dyslexic person. I would like to dedicate this book to my family and close friends. They are the ones that had to deal with the emotional roller coaster of watching me go through life with dyslexia.

I will never forget the tears in my mom's eyes when someone tried to stick me in the back corner of society, where I could not hurt anyone. Writing this book has forced me to spill my insides out on the table, sorting through them, and hoping to make some sense of them. My goal is to help others understand what it is like to be dyslexic, and to help other dyslexic people discover they are not alone. After completing this book I hope to overcome the hurt and anger, I wish not to tie up my present life by my past. There has been much soul searching and painful memories revisited.

I apologize if I have forgotten anyone that has helped me through this process. Also, I would like to add that I do not want to hold grudges against anyone that did not understand or used my dyslexia to attack me. Those were bitter feelings caused by my pain, which you will feel reading this book. I feel sorry for them and truly believe they fear any learning disorder can be transmitted like the common cold. Maybe they do not want to think the human body can have problems and not be perfect, or possibly they fear the unknown.

Humans have always pushed aside things that are not the norms, as is the case with dyslexics. Lucky for me, my friends and family have helped me fight this "classifying." That is why I do not think it has been as hard on me as it has been on them. Since I have always lived with it, I know no different. I thank them for standing by me through losing a job to flunking a class, or listening to others make fun of my reading and writing. I have learned from them and God that I am no better or worse than anyone else. With their help, I am going to burst out of any stereotype and overcome anything put before me. For all the family, friends, and teachers that have helped, thank you; I love you all!

Chapter 1

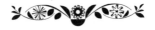

A statement I once read sums up my purpose and desire for writing this book: "What I kept, I lost; what I spent, I had; and what I gave, I have." My hope is to provide an understanding of dyslexia—and living with it—to everyone who reads this book. In return, I hope to understand more about myself and hopefully set free some ghosts that have haunted me. These ghosts will appear throughout the book. Consequently, I feel our true immortality is to pass the lessons we have learned to others. Jon Locke put it best, "The improvement of understanding is for two ends: first, our own increase of knowledge; secondly, to enable us to deliver that know-ledge to others." My giving of this gift of knowledge cost me great pain as I relived my memories and lessons, as you will soon read and hopefully understand. But I believe it is worth it.

What is dyslexia? The scientific term for dyslexia is: "Dyslexia, or more properly, functional dyslexia or language disorder is a neurological dysfunction affecting visual, auditory and spatial perception." The most commonly publicized aspects of dyslexia have been the perceptual problems associated with reading and language disorders, but dyslexia is much more than this. Dyslexia involves a wide range of perceptual difficulties in which information from the body's sensors arrives to the brain in a mixed or confused state. Individuals suffering from dyslexia may experience confusion of time and space, visual perception challenges, auditory understanding problems, left-right disorientation, and difficulty learning days of the week or months of the year. After reading this scientific term, you might be thinking one of these thoughts: one, dyslexia is what I have, or two, someone I know has dyslexia. A third thought might be, how in the world did Girard ever write this book with that over his head? I hope to write this book from all viewpoints, painting a complete picture of what it is like to be dyslexic.

I prefer a brief and short definition of dyslexia. My definition is that a dyslexic person has trouble processing data from the senses of the body dealing with two-dimensional (2-D) items, and yet has exceptional talent processing three-dimensional (3-D) items. A good example of a 2-D difficulty would be hearing and recognizing an unfamiliar word. The word enters the brain and is unclear to the dyslexic person until it is repeated, developing a clear footprint in the brain. An explanation of 3-D, according to the National Health and Welfare Department, is that dyslexic people have above-average intelligence and superior abilities manipulating 3-D symbols. This includes art, math reasoning, abstract reasoning, building, mechanical items, and seeing the whole picture. Unfortunately, current testing and learning policies in schools only measure 2-D IQs in students.

With the definition out of the way, now I can start explaining what it was, and is, like to live as a dyslexic person. My first feeling of being different from other children was the process of remembering and repeating new, unfamiliar words. Other children could do this easily, while I stumbled and tripped, giving everyone the illusion that I was slow or lazy. Looking back, it seemed to me that my mind only consisted of long-term memory. I was only capable of repeating something new after it had been engraved in my mind.

For years I pronounced my oldest sister's name, "Delray," as "Duray." I started confusing words (for example "tornado" instead of "tomato" and "baby gun" for "BB gun"). I would ask for a tornado for dinner and mean tomato. One night this problem scared my mother and reddened my bottom. My mom was deathly afraid of lightning storms, and would distract herself by keeping busy cooking for the family. On one such occasion, she was cooking dinner and asked us what we wanted for dinner. The sky was dark and gray outside, and the wind was howling through the door only as it can on the treeless plains of North Dakota. Water was seeping in under the door from the strong rain and wind. The lightning was flashing, with thunder shaking the house seconds later, letting us know it was hitting the ground close to our house. "Tornado, tornado, tornado!" I yelled, meaning I wanted tomatoes for dinner. My mom rushed us to the basement for cover as fast as she could, only to learn I meant tomato. I received a spanking and never touched or asked for a tomato for years after that.

Most kids outgrow this phase, but for a dyslexic child it followed me throughout my life. Maybe this is my true inner child—the child locked inside us all—as so many books talk about these days. Unfortunately, I still confuse words today, which drives my friends crazy.

The pain of the backside never came close to the pain of the heart, and so it was with switching the words BB gun for baby gun. My Uncle Elmer gave me a BB gun for my fifth birthday. I really liked Uncle Elmer and still feel bad today for embarrassing him. It was at a Sunday afternoon family function. Everyone was sitting around the table eating, including another uncle, who I disliked and with whom Elmer had experienced a long family feud. The less favored uncle asked me what kind of gun I had gotten. The room grew silent. My mom's eyes met mine as she placed more food on the table. She was hoping that I could say it right this time. I thought to myself, "This time I am going to say it right. He is not going to make a fool of Uncle Elmer and me. I will show him I can say it." Unfortunately, "baby gun" came out of my mouth. The obnoxious uncle's family members all cackled like Cinderella's repulsive sisters when she wanted to attend the ball. My asinine uncle had always made fun of my speech, but he now ran it into the ground by hitting on Elmer's nerve. After that I stopped talking around large groups.

Elbert Hubbard put it best, "He who does not understand your silence will probably not understand your words." I became silent in groups, not because I did not have anything to say, but because I was afraid of what would come out of my mouth. One too many times in the past I had stumbled on reading or repeating an unfamiliar word in a public group. If felt like I was trying to get the word out of my mouth after someone had stuck it to the roof with peanut butter. I would stop trying after the third time and hang my head in shame. Like Cinderella, I outgrew the negative thinking of my relatives, no longer spending time with them as I grew older. Thank God for the reinforcement of the positive thoughts my sister Noreen would give me at these difficult times in my life.

My speech and writing challenges have always been used as ammunition against me, as in the incident with my uncle. My relatives never understood my dyslexia. I have learned that things not understood or different are often considered evil or dysfunctional. Since I was not a bad child, I was looked at as different and, therefore, dumb. Those misinformed relatives would even talk to me slowly, loudly, and even baby-talked. They would argue with my mom that they thought I was slow. Luckily for me, my mom never gave up or listened to them. Also, she endowed me with an unusual first name. My unique name caused people to stumble while pronouncing it. This taught me at an early age that most people cannot say every word correctly and no one is perfect. I found that people seemed to have problems pronouncing my name, yet everything else was easy for them to pronounce. Unfortunately, it was not that way for me. Funny how life works out sometimes!

My mom, as many mothers of dyslexic children do, became discouraged. She was frustrated with the early signs of dyslexia as they began to emerge. Not understanding what dyslexia was, she did not know how to help. The slow process of learning simple tasks, such as tying my shoes, frustrated my mom even more. Her temper grew short because I did not learn to tie my shoes quickly like my two sisters who had learned to tie their shoes at an early age. In her frustration, Mom would send me to my room, spank me, ground me from TV, not let me go outside to play, or use any other punishment she could think of. She eventually refused to tie my shoes for me, not knowing that this added stress made matters worse. Finally, I learned to tie my shoes with help from my sister, Noreen. I think she felt sorry for me, or got tired of tying my shoes. Noreen worked with me each morning and night using a song (the one about the rabbit and the hole). You hold the shoe strings up in the air, then pick one string as the rabbit and sing: "The rabbit goes around the bent tree (which is the other string), the tree makes a rabbit ear, the rabbit runs around the tree, goes back through the hole, and makes two rabbit ears." This kind of association method works well for dyslexic children, since it requires the use of more than one sense. For years I would say the poem as I tied my shoes and it worked. Tying my shoes eventually became a habit. This is important to a dyslexic child—repeating a process until it becomes a habit. It is the best way I know to overcome any of my dyslexic disabilities.

Looking back now, another noticeable dyslexic trait was my ability to disassemble mechanical items throughout the house, and then put them back together. Dyslexic people have strong mechanical and technical skills. I could take a flashlight apart, then use the battery, light bulb, and a piece of wire to make the bulb light up outside the flashlight. This was accomplished before I was old enough to start school. It is important for a dyslexic child to have building blocks, Legos, and other 3-D toys to help them grow.

If my mom asked me to do something, I would become confused, unorganized, and disoriented—more signs of dyslexia. Yet, I could disassemble my toys and then reassemble them. When a flashlight went out, a toaster went on the blink, a clock stopped ticking, or any household item stopped working, I could usually make it work. This also confused my parents, but even more confusing to them was that I could assemble my Christmas toys by studying the pictures on the directions. My mom could not understand how I could build things easily, yet have difficulty speaking. It was as if my hands had a superior connection to my brain, leaving little room for my speech. It was my flashlight accomplishment that helped Mom believe in me. Her belief in me helped direct my life to more positive outcomes. To this day, when I go home to visit my mom, she will have a list of items she needs fixed. It was hard for me to understand—if I were so dumb— why other people could not figure out things I considered simple.

Another indication of dyslexia is messiness, and I was always messy. My shirt would be backwards or untucked, and it took my mom and two sisters to keep me cleaned up and in order. It was years before I overcame my bad dressing habits.

I remember standing in a store once when my mom grabbed me, twisted and adjusted my clothing and hair, trying to make me look presentable. They always told me, "You are the messiest kid I have ever seen." Since then I have talked to mothers of dyslexic children and found this characteristic to be common Mom must have been really frustrated with me as a child, since she is a very neat person. Because of my slow learning and disorderly appearance, people perceived me as lazy and slow. This is how most dyslexic people appear to the outside world. Dyslexics are seen as those who do what they want: take toys apart, not learn daily functions (such as tying shoes), and in a constant state of confusion to the outside world.

I was the youngest of three children. Two older sisters (who looked out for their younger brother), a mom, a dad, cats, dogs, sheep, chickens, and some geese all called our place home on the windy prairie plains of North Dakota. My dad was a truck driver and mom worked at home with us kids. I thought life was grand. Each day I would wake up, go outside, and eat fresh vegetables or straw-berries from the garden in the summer. In the winter I would build snow forts and play with the family pets. My all-time favorite pastime was lying on my back in the deep green grass. Using a sheep as a pillow, I would watch the soft, fluffy clouds roll by as only they can in North Dakota. All good things do end and so did my fairy tale childhood.

Inside the mind of a dyslexic, the thought process is in perpetual fast motion. My mind was always racing to think up practical jokes to play on my sisters or ways to improve my bike's performance. Unfortunately, it did not help me to master the skills of reading. My mother eventually gave up trying to teach me reading and writing. I was constantly reminded of my inabilities by my mother's remarks. When she was asked to give me extra help at home, she would respond, "That is why I send him to school. That is their job."

For me, the feeling of being disoriented became stronger while in Dickinson, North Dakota. In the first grade, as I tried to develop basic reading and writing skills, the school system discovered my learning problem. (I use the word "discovered," because during my whole life I have tried to hide my dyslexia, at all costs, as if it were an embarrassing family secret. I would let people think anything— that I was lazy, dumb, etc.—anything but the dark truth. People more easily accept you if they have the illusion that you chose your behavior, rather than you have no choice in your actions. Only now do I openly tell people about my dyslexia). The school system decided I was slow, but did not diagnose dyslexia. They had drawn their own conclusions about my learning disability.

My mother always made weekly trips into town with the family pickup, a red 1952 Chevy. It made much noise as she tried to shift it into gear, but not as much noise as she made yelling at it. The gears would grind each time she would push the lever into the next gear. Then she would yell obscenities that not even the cats were called when they sneaked into the house. I always accompanied her to town for the weekly shopping trip for groceries, but one week the routine was different. She dressed me up in my Sunday clothes—the one shirt and pants I could never wear unless we were going to church. Mom was acting different. I stood there as she straightened my shirt and pants into place, like she always did after I dressed myself. She gave them a pull and a tug, as if I were a sack of flour and as if she were mad at me. I became frightened as she grew consistently short tempered with me. I then knew how the old red truck felt.

A favorite pastime of my sister's was playing jokes on me. One of her favorite jokes was to convince me that I was adopted and could be returned if I misbehaved. I was not adopted, but it worked to manipulate me for my sister's needs. On this trip to town, I thought I was being returned to the adoption agency for a more suitable brother. Then I became deeply frightened. I did everything my mom asked, but she was still frustrated with me. I physically attached myself to her as we walked around the house preparing to go to town. Once in town, I stayed attached to my mom in each store we entered. On previous trips I would usually drift off into my own world, lose her, and run around in a panic trying to find her. This time though, I did not leave her side. I had tears in my eyes, because I could sense something was deadly wrong.

Little did I know it was my first day of school, and my mom felt she was losing her little boy. Our last stop was the school. We walked into a large building and mom sat me down in a strange room full of kids I had never seen before. She told me to stay there until my sister Noreen came to get me. Together we would walk to the bus. I never knew there were so many children my age. As my mother walked away with tears in her eyes, I watched with tears in my eyes. I ran after her, only to be pushed back into my seat. Here I was, with no idea for how long. The fear almost killed me, and I started crying frantically. Was this the adoption place my sister had told me about? Would I ever see my mom and dad again? Who was this strange lady in the front of the room telling me not to cry anymore?

I finally realized what was going on as this new lady, my first grade teacher. (Kindergarten was provided), explained who she was and what we were doing there. My endless play days were gone. This was the first day of the rest of my life, during which I would have to be some place each school or working day. The only unstructured time that remained was my summer vacation, and even that would be taken away after I started working in my later years. I made it through the day and waited for my sister to meet me. Today I can still feel the fear as I wondered if my sister would come for me. It felt like years before she got there. I was never so glad to see her in all my life. Maybe that is why I hate waiting for people even now. I will drive to someone's house instead of having them come over, just so I do not have to wait for them.

By now you are thinking, what does this have to do with dyslexia and where is he going with this? I never did like my first grade teacher, and she had her hands full with a child who had lived outside most of his life, doing whatever he wanted. Having been a true free spirit, this was the first time I had to go by rules; no talking, no walking around, and asking to go to the bathroom. I remember my rear end hurting each night from sitting so long on those wooden chairs. The discovery of my learning disability was this first grade teacher's ticket to get me out of her class and her life. In my adult life I crossed paths with another teacher who explained to me that she did not get paid enough to teach "children with problems." I always wondered if this was the attitude my first grade teacher had.

My school year had reached the point of my first teacher's conference. I can remember the events as if they happened yesterday. Noreen and I were riding along in the family truck, listening to my mother grind the gears. We visited Noreen's teacher first. Noreen and I stayed outside the classroom, watching our mom sit on the other side of the desk from the teacher. I thought what power teachers have; my mother listened closely to every word. Little did I know just how much power a teacher has over a young one's future life. My mom sat there nodding her head as the teacher talked. Finally, my mom gave her an okay, smiled, and walked out of the room. We followed her downstairs to see my teacher, since it was now my turn.

As we approached the classroom, I could see a somber group of people in the room. My mom entered the classroom and the door was closed. Immediately, panic rushed through my body. Why was my conference so different from Noreen's? I paced back and forth in front of the closed classroom door. It was not just my teacher sitting in there with my mom. It was also the principal, vice principal, and another man I did not recognize. Noreen announced to me that something was wrong. "What have you done?" she yelled at me. Again, I experienced the fear of being sent to the orphanage and being placed for adoption. I could see now that everyone was yelling at my mom and she had started to cry. The only thing I could remember, that I might have done wrong, was the time I pushed a kid down on the playground because he took something from me. Noreen was upset with me for making our mother cry. My mom jumped up from the chair and ran out of the room, with tears running down her face, and her eyes red from crying. As she came through the door, she grabbed Noreen and me, pulled us down the hall out to the red truck, and recklessly drove home. She cried all the way home, not saying a word. No one spoke, and I felt sick. I must have done something terrible, but it was just dyslexia.

As we arrived home and pulled into the gravel driveway, my mom dashed out of the truck and ran into the house, leaving Noreen and me alone in the truck. My sister hit my side, encouraging me to open the door. She pushed me out onto the gravel surface and I scraped my hand. I recall this incident anytime I scrape my hand, and memories of that pain floods my mind. That was the last I saw of my mother that day. I knew whatever I had done was bad, and now I looked at my bleeding hand and realized no one would clean it for me. Noreen walked slowly into the house and I was alone, lying in the driveway bleeding. The pickup was facing north. I was wearing a yellow shirt with white stripes and jeans two sizes too big so I could grow into them. The sun was setting, and not a sound could be heard except my heart beating with fear.

I slowly got up, went into the house where my oldest sister, Delray, had just discovered my mortal sin—I had made our mother cry. In my family it was the worst of all evils. My dad was also upset. We usually got away with many things, only to be yelled at. Delray was now standing in front of me, then she pushed me to the floor and started screaming at me. My father walked in and I knew I was going to die. I had done the worst thing in my life and he was going to kill me. Delray informed him that I had made our mother cry. He gave me the look of death, the look that only a parent can give their child. Never before had I been so scared. I was beyond the point of being afraid, because I knew I was going to be sent to the orphanage (if lucky). Fortunately for me, dad passed me by and went into my parents' bedroom where my mom was still crying. Delray restrained me to the floor, making sure I was accessible to my father when he returned. To our surprise, he returned and told her to release me. Then he walked over to a chair and sat. His face was expressionless and blank. I had not died, except in my father's heart.

Delray uncuffed my hands from her grip and walked into the kitchen to join Noreen. Laying on the floor across the room from my dad, I could still hear my mother crying. She would almost stop crying and then would start all over. My sisters went to the bedroom that they shared, and stayed the rest of the night. Dad stared at the wall, with no expression on his face. Before this day we had a great relationship. He would take me with him in the truck or bring me things. Everything was great before this, but afterwards when he talked to me, he had the look that said, "My only son is dumb. He will never be normal."

My father and I did not talk much after that or do anything together unless instructed by Mom. He would play with other kids, but he would tell me to go away if I tried to join in. Dad could never look at me straight in the eye unless he was really mad. I knew he felt that he had placed a bad seed in the world, and could not look at me because I was a reminder of that. On his death bed I was the only family member he would not talk to. He never told me he loved me. I was not perfect, and because of that I embarrassed him. Everyone in that small northern town knew which kids had to go to special reading classes and everyone knew it was his kid, Girard. I do not want to make my dad sound bad. He was a great man and did whatever he could for his family. My dad did not get to see me graduate from college, get my first good job, receive my Masters in business, or write this book. It really hurts me deeply that I cannot show him how wrong everyone was about his son.

We did not eat that night. I just got up and went to bed by myself. As I lay in bed, looking up at the sky, I cried so hard I could feel the pillow growing wet as the tears ran down my face. My chest hurt from the pain I had given my family. Praying to God, I asked Him to come and take me to His place, where I could go and not hurt anybody. I cried as only someone truly alone in the world can cry, with every part of my body and soul. Then a white warming light seemed to appear in my room above my head. I slowly drifted off to sleep.

Now I am close to God, and His strength and unconditional love have helped me through many tough times. I found out later that the school system had diagnosed me as mentally retarded; because I was unable to function and read with the rest of the children in my class. They strongly felt I should be institutionalized so I could get special help. In

1968 I do not think the special help would have been anything more than drugs to control me and a special room. I might still be sitting there today, or living as a homeless person after the government cut funding in the 1980's, unable to read or speak effectively after years of special treatment. Thank God my mom said no and fought for me. I am glad she had the will power to do so.

Fortunately my family was not confronted with this decision two years earlier, because both my parents had to be hospitalized. My dad had developed a tumor on his spine that collapsed two of his vertebrae. The surgeon used one of his ribs and four steel bolts to reconstruct a new vertebra. Dad was the second person in the world to ever have this kind of back surgery. Because of the complexity of the operation he could not move for 90 days while the bones healed into place. Therefore, he lay in a hospital bed on what looked to me like two ironing boards, one on his front and one his back. The nurses would turn him every few minutes to prevent fluids from accumulating in his lungs. In those days, children under 12 were not allowed to visit. This included me. After the 90 days and a lengthy recuperation period, my father went back to school and received his GED and Associate degree in accounting. My mom, not to be outdone by my dad, simultaneously became ill and had a hysterectomy.

While both parents were hospitalized, Noreen, who is five years my senior, was forced to care for me. This mothering necessity carried on throughout my life. Even today, I am very close to her. My older sister, Delray, was in high school at the time of my parents illnesses. She worked at a local fruit stand to feed the family (I guess I owe my sisters a great big thanks). These hard times are not talked about among my family members.

Chapter 2

My mother decided to transfer me to another elementary school across town. At this point in my life I viewed the outside world as a place where they: (1) stuck you in beds for three months (like my dad), (2) yelled at you and made you cry (like my mom), or (3) disliked you and thought you were dumb (like me). It was at this time I met the first non-family member who would change all of that. My new elementary school teacher gave me hope. She was dedicated and was not one to quickly stick people into categories just to save time and energy. My heart goes out to families that have had a family member wrongfully judged and institutionalized. It is a sad loss to society.

My new teacher spent quality time helping me. Sadly, I can only picture her face, but I cannot remember her name. Thinking back now, her loving and caring manner influenced me in so many ways. I even look for her qualities in the ladies I date. These qualities were displayed when she spent extra time helping me with my alphabet while the other children played outside. When I did well she would pat the top of my head or hug me. I will never forget the feeling of the warmth in her arms. The warm feeling I received from her hugs was something I needed then. Her hand seemed to say, "You have done well," instead of the hand of so many teachers that said, "You have done wrong." Our society acknowledges only bad behavior and expects good behavior to happen without acknowledgement.

I strongly encourage anyone who has or works with a dyslexic child to reinforce them for good behavior or accomplishments. The world will do the scolding. I usually make this comment to each teacher I meet, "You have a great job. Each day you can make a difference in someone's life and that difference could change the world tomorrow, for good or bad. Most people spend their lives in a job that makes other people financially wealthier." I get many answers back from that statement, but few have said that was why they decided to become a teacher.

Apparently this was the reason my first grade teacher was teaching. She worked diligently with my problem of differentiating between the letters "b" and "d", and troubles I had remembering which way the letters "s" and "n" faced. I could not understand how other children could hear or look at a word once and then spell it aloud. This confused me since I was unable to perform this task. I would get mixed up and become confused with my reading and writing skills. In class, the word "Pam" was on our spelling test. It seems so easy now, but it gave me much trouble then. I would spend hours working on that word, sorting the letters in my brain. It seemed to me that when I would just about get it right, someone would jump into my brain and scramble the letters around again like a puzzle. I stared at the name tag of a classmate whose name was Pam, because I knew it was on the next spelling test (each person's name was on the wall behind the teacher). Not listening to what the teacher was saying, I focused on repeating the letters P, A, M, in my mind. I became upset with myself, resolving not to make my mom cry again by having my new teacher yell at her during a teacher's conference. The test came and I passed, but I got the word "Pam" wrong. I spelled it "Pma." I tried hard for my mom's sake, and because I secretly liked the young classmate named Pam.

The next year my family moved to Valley City, North Dakota. After graduating from college, my dad found a job as an accountant with a plumbing firm. This move was a stroke of good luck for me. Valley City was the home of one of North Dakota's teachers colleges. The college provided the local elementary school system with student teachers. These student teachers could give me the extra attention I needed. Being fresh in the field, the student teachers were energetic about teaching and, better yet, they were being graded on their skills.

From day one in Valley City I started those oh-so-fun special reading classes. I was elected to attend the reading class because I had a low SAT score. As a member of the special reading group, I was required to leave the classroom at a scheduled time of the day. I would watch the clock and hope the teacher would forget to dismiss me. This was the part of the day I hated most . . . experiencing the feeling of not being good enough to sit with the rest of my class. Some of my teachers would announce to the class, "Would the students who need to leave with Ms. White, please meet her in the back of the room." Other teachers were not as considerate and would just say, "Would the children with learning problems please follow Ms. White out of the room," or they would use the term "slower readers." This was not as mentally damaging as the other children who whispered "Will the dumb ones leave" or "Hey stupid, time for your idiot class." Ashamed, I would walk out of the room, becoming numb to what was said. I would then be joined by other members of the special group. As we walked slowly past the other students, we would hang our heads in shame. It felt as if we were being sentenced to death, going to meet our Maker. Our time had come and the death sentence was about to be carried out. The teacher would pause from the lesson until we had left the room. We all met at the door and followed another teacher into the hall. As we walked silently down the hall, we hoped to not be noticed by children in other classrooms. This would expose our secret.

The group met for an hour in any available room—locker room, empty classrooms, gym, teacher's lounge, or janitor's closet. The special reading group teacher worked with us, using new-found skills learned in college. We often felt we were guinea pigs.

The student teachers came up with a wide range of answers to my reading problem. Initially, they thought I had astigmatism and gave me reading glasses that, of course, did not help. I was tested and retested until I was finally diagnosed with dyslexia in the third grade. Today, I laugh about all the different methods or new tricks the school system used on me. They tried records, slides, cassettes, summer school, coloring books, flash cards, films, and one year they got me a special desk. I could sit off to the side from the rest of my classmates and not be disturbed. The desk had high walls so no one could see me or I them. My class work consisted of listening to tapes, which were from the rest of the class's homework. It was embarrassment at its best. I would work on learning items that I should have learned years before, but had instead confused me.

It was exciting to see what new learning toys or games the school system would purchase each year, as they tried to find that one magical teaching tool that was going to help me perform like the rest of the class. I made my own game of it, trying to figure out how to work the new toys before the student teacher could figure out how to work them. Today I am still very analytical. This is another characteristic of being dyslexic. Maybe it is a survival tool, such as one who is blind and learns to hear better than the sighted person. Most of the teaching tools sold to the school system never seemed to work well. The best solution for most learning problems was one-on-one time.

In a way, the special classes could be fun because I was with other children who had something in common with me. There were two parts of the special reading class I really hated and could not enjoy, no matter how hard I tried. One was walking out of the classroom for the special group meetings. The feeling I had was something I call the "Rudolph the Red Nose Reindeer" syndrome. When the mud fell off Rudolph's nose, everyone teased him. The second part I despised was having a teacher or student teacher who really did not care, and view me as an inconvenience to them. One such student teacher was assigned to my group.

The school was short on classrooms and, being last on the needs list, we met in a janitor's closet. The small makeshift classroom smelled of cigarette smoke and cleaning fluids. It was filled with mops, brooms, and other janitorial supplies. The five desks were placed in a circle, with the student teacher in the middle. As this student teacher used his new-found authority, he would turn on his heel and call on one of us to read. He was a football player who had decided to become a teacher, for lack of anything better to do with his football scholarship. We would sit in our circle and read aloud, each person taking a turn. The teacher drew close to our faces, waiting for the first mispronounced word. When a student stumbled on a word, the teacher's face grew red and tense, and his lips pursed as his eyes pinched together. This is how he told us, in a nonverbal way, not to miss another word. When a word was missed a second time, his hands would come crashing down on the desk top. On the third mistake, he grabbed us by our throats. The more we missed a word, the louder his voice became. At times he would grab us, pulling us out of our chairs, and shake our bodies like rag dolls.

One day, my turn came to read and the student before me had missed a word three times, already making the student teacher mad. Then I was having trouble reading a word. The word just seemed to keep scrambling on me. The harder I tried, the madder the teacher became. He was yelling by then. I could see by the faces of the other children that they were glad it was me his anger was pointed at, and not them. I kept trying to say the word, but I could not do it. He started yelling and pounding his fists on my desk and said, "You're going to be able to read it. You don't want to know what is going to happen to you if you can't." He grabbed me. It hurt, and now my heart was beating fast. I was really scared and could feel tears coming down my face. But I made no sound or movement, hoping not to upset him anymore. I could see the other children were afraid for me and of what he might do next. We had never seen him this upset before. He walked to the janitor's desk and picked up a pair of scissors. "Okay. One last time. What is the word, Girard?", he said as he moved closer to me. I tried and tried, but I still could not pronounce it right. He then took the scissors, sharp end down, and lunged them toward my hand. All I saw was a streak of silver coming for me and quickly moved my hand out of the way. The scissors just missed my hand, piercing into the desk top where my hand had been seconds before.

Now I was frightened for my life. Should I run? Should I cry? I was shocked that he really wanted to hurt me. Waiting for his next move, I realized my life would never be safe with anybody. He grabbed the scissors, which now stuck in the desk top, and pulled with a violent yank. The tip of the scissors broke off and remained imbedded in the wooden desk top. That could have been my hand. The teacher then grabbed me and pulled me out of my seat. He held me two feet in the air, looking eye-to-eye with me. I had no idea what he was going to do. The only thing I could feel was one of my shoes falling off as I hung in midair. A button popped off my new shirt, and I later got spanked because I refused to tell my mom how it happened. To this day, she does not know what happened. If there was ever a time in my life I felt I was looking in the eye of the devil, this was it. His mouth opened and sewer gas rolled out, carrying the words, "Now look what you made me do. This is all your fault." He then tossed me back into my chair as he gained some composure, and walked around the circle yelling words which made no sense to me. I was still crying, which seemed to upset him again. The teacher grabbed me, but paused and changed his mind, throwing me back into my seat. Then he kicked the door open and left the room. I sat and cried. Finally, my fellow group members comforted me and I could stop crying. We walked back to the classroom and slowly took our seats. The teacher stopped her lecture when she spotted my red eyes and torn shirt. I looked as if I were returning from battle, and I had lost. After being asked about my appearance and the location of the student teacher, we told her what happened. The student teacher who attacked me was not allowed to teach again, and had to switch his major. This was probably fortunate for many students out there who could not move their hands as fast as I could.

Another teacher I did not like and never forgot was an older teacher who gave me a hard time because she did not understand my learning problem. She was frustrated since she could not teach me as well as the other students. Consequently, she treated me like a second-rate individual. I was viewed as the problem child, the pain in her side. As you can tell, I still have no love for this lady or her teaching skills. A good example of how she felt about me was the time I was playing on the playground and broke my nose. I was playing with the other special group members at recess. We stuck together because of our common bond, and since we were considered uncool. While we were playing, a log fell on my nose. My nose was broken and it started to bleed. I went into the classroom where the teacher was sitting behind her desk, and asked her what I should do. The blood was flowing over the saturated towels in my hand. She quickly looked up and scowled, telling me I was getting blood on the floor and to go to the bathroom. She then went back to the papers she was working on. I walked to the bathroom and let the blood from my nose run into the sink. The bleeding did not stop or even slow, causing great pain to my face. I could feel my heart beating in my bleeding nose. My nose bled as I stood alone in the bathroom throughout the remainder of recess. I thought I heard the sound of water dripping, but it was the blood from my nose dripping in the sink. The teacher sent a student to get me when class started. I went back to the classroom still bleeding, and was told to go home. As I walked the seven blocks home, a trail of blood followed. By the time I got home, my mom had to hold me up so I would not pass out from the loss of blood. Then I was taken to the hospital. After returning home, I stayed out of school for a few days. Again, my mom went to the school to defend my honor.

After that incident, the teacher was even more impatient with me and refused to call on me in class. I would hold my hand up and she would not call on me to answer questions. Once, I just kept my hand up to see how long it would take to be called upon. My hand was in the air for 15 minutes. Finally, the teacher looked at me and said "What?" I gave my answer and she responded with, "That was 15 minutes ago, why are you answering that now?" I simply said, "It took you that long to call on me." Then I stopped listening to her and did a wide range of other things, including making bows out of wire and rubber bands, and using toothpicks as arrows. The other special group members and I would shoot them into the false ceiling. We would also take a new pen and start writing one, two, three, etc., to see who could write the most numbers before the pen ran out of ink. It would fill a notebook. Most of these self-entertaining activities were ignored by the teacher.

Once, I took blackboard chalk, rubbed it on my hands, and clapped them together, making it look like a cloud of smoke. This upset the teacher and she went into a long speech about how I was so dumb for doing that and asked, "What is wrong with you?" I would not have remembered this incident, except that the school had two classes for each grade. The teacher for the other class had been teaching her students about the Watergate scandal. Unknown to my teacher, they had taped our class. This was all recorded and the other class listened to it. The students informed me that their teacher told them this was not right, and my teacher should have not said those things to me. The other teacher turned the tape in to the principal's office and my teacher became even less tolerant toward me. I began to hurt more for my mother than for me. The son she cared for had all these problems and she could not help him, although she was an ex-teacher herself. Kids teasing me, she could understand, but not the teachers or other adults.

It was in this class I aced an algebra test, and most of the rest of the class flunked. While dyslexic people face difficulties in some areas, they usually have above-average intelligence, and great mathematical and reasoning skills. My strong math ability helps me today in the computer field. After passing the test and seeing the teacher's reaction, I knew I was going to get in trouble. I could not understand why. My teacher always wanted me to do better and I had really tried hard. Now she was yelling at the rest of the class for doing worse than me—the dumb one. She said,"He is supposed to get this grade, but not the rest of you." Those words shocked me. I thought she wanted me to do well, but I found out that people do not like someone doing better or worse than they perceive you are capable of. She was really mad, yelling at the students that they had always done well. They were crying and this upset her. She stormed out of the class and slammed the door behind her. We all just looked at each other. Soon the other students were yelling at me for upsetting the teacher. I knew what faced me after school. The teacher had set the tone for me to be the punching bag to take their anger out on.

When it started to get out of hand, the teacher ran back in. I was happy to see her, thinking she was the least of two evils, but I was wrong. She approached my desk, grabbed me by my arm, and pulled me from my chair. I fell down, almost hitting the floor, then she jerked me up to my feet. I had no idea what I had done, and could not believe what she was saying, or should I say yelling. "You cheated, didn't you? Someone helped you! You can't get that grade . . . tell me!" I was really scared now and could feel her fingernails digging into my skin. Her fingernails left marks in my skin for the rest of the day. All I could say was "No." It was hard to talk with the lump in my throat. Then she jerked me down the hall to the principal's office. Just before we went in, she released her death grip. Giving me one last push on the back to let me know she could still hurt me if needed. I was instructed to sit in the detention chair. Then she left the room. I was crying now, trying not to make a sound, and just looking at the floor. The principal asked me if I had cheated on the test and I said no. In a soft voice, he told me to just sit there until I felt better, then he would take me back to class. I made sure never to ace a test again, and I would purposely get some wrong because that is what they wanted. The cost of doing bad was less than doing good. Never again did I do anything outstanding until college, where a teacher again accused me of cheating.

After the principal returned me to my classroom, I sat in the class not saying a word. After class, I slowly walked home thinking of my day in hell, until some classmates jumped me. They beat me up for making them look bad in school that day. An older man came out of his house and stopped them. I finally made it home, with my face hurting, my heart hurting, and my clothing dirty from being forced down in the dirt. I had a general all-over pain. My mom met me at the door, since my teacher had called. After seeing my dirty clothes and hearing my explanation of what had happened, she sent me to my room. I was only allowed to leave my room for supper. Noreen was the only one who came in to see me, so I explained everything to her. She gave me a hug that made it seem better, because someone believed me. Again that night, I cried until the white light of God put me to sleep.

Dyslexics are often not given the opportunity to develop strengths because we are working so hard to overcome our weaknesses. This leads to the game of "What if?" We have been dealt the cards and we are at this point in our life. I end up thinking that I just have to go on, because I can only control what is ahead of me.

I found that in life, work, school, friendships, and relationships, your peers will punish you for behavior that causes you to stand out. Unfortunately, with dyslexia, I stand out each day. I have now learned to live with it, but that year was one of the toughest for being picked on by my classmates. It became socially acceptable once the teacher had done it.

I was also teased for my unique pen grip. Most dyslexics have difficulty with writing, and have an unusual pen grip to compensate, forming letters and numbers in unusual ways.

My pen grip was the butt of many jokes. Again, I do not want to sound negative, but it is reality. My mother would tell me, "If somebody teases you, just ignore them." Well, that is hard. The teasing would range from being beaten up or chased home, to having my homework stolen, or being pushed off my bike and having my bike taken. I stopped riding my bike to school after getting it back, because my mom had purchased the bike with money she received from being in a bad car accident. She informed me that she would not go through that again to get me another bike. I was beaten up at least twice a year until we moved away from Valley City.

I do not want to sound like every teacher I had was wicked, or that I hate the teaching profession. If it had not been for a special group of teachers, who really cared about me and took the time to help, I would have never made it. So, I owe a lot to them.

One of these teachers was Mr. Baltimore, my sixth grade teacher. He really helped by giving me my self-confidence. For the first time I felt I could do something. I ran track in sixth grade and won six ribbons—more than anyone else. Mr. Baltimore asked if he could give my ribbons to me in class. I had no idea why until the next day. He called out the other students' names, who then walked up and took their ribbons. He called on me last. One ribbon at a time, I would walk up to get it, and sit back down. Then he would call me up for the next ribbon. After it was over, Mr. Baltimore said something that has stuck with me for the rest of my life, and helped me in times of trouble: "Each day I see this class making fun of Girard for his reading skills, but today he has outdone all of you in running, and he's not making fun of you for being a slow runner." The class was still and no one said a word. I always tried to do well in track for Mr. Baltimore, and almost went to state in high school until a double hernia stopped me.

My guardian angel of a teacher, who had defended me, also helped me to learn to read by memorization. He knew about dyslexia and helped me to read by memorizing shapes. Most words have a unique shape to them. Take my name, Girard. Close your eyes to the point that they are almost shut. You can see the high shape of the "G", the "r" pointing to the right, and the tall "d" at the end. As you can see, this makes a unique shape, like tracing a circle around the word. The shape recognition does not always work well. For instance, the words "from" and "form" are too much alike, and I always get them mixed up. If I glance at a word, read it aloud, and mistake it for a wrong word, it is embarrassing when I am corrected by others. Because of the embarrassment, I have been forced to make light of the situation.

In Mr. Baltimore's class, I started passing spelling tests with his help. After acing my first spelling test, he gave me a candy bar, and had the whole class stand up to applaud for me. I turned red, because I was so used to the other side of the coin. It was especially rewarding to look over at the young lady I had a secret crush on and watch her applaud enthusiastically for me. Mr. Baltimore left an everlasting impression on me. I learned that: Yes, I can do it and yes, I can get the applause I need as I achieve accomplishments in life. I do not want to make it sound like I do well for the applause, but many things I do not really do for myself. My purpose for achievement is more for my family who supported me, to show them that I can do anything I want. I want my family and teachers who helped me to be proud of me, so they know they did make a difference in the world.

While in school, I broke my right arm. This turned out to be a good thing. Another prominent characteristic of dyslexia is the inability to distinguish between right and left. Using my broken arm as a tool to determine direction, I could resolve my left-right confusion. From that point on, I could distinguish my left from my right. I knew how to write from left to right and turn left or right while walking. All I had to remember was which arm I broke. The other benefit of breaking my arm was since I was right-handed, my teacher would do all my writing for me while the other students did their work. He not only wrote down the answer, but questioned me when I gave him the wrong answer.

The one big influence outside school that helped me with my dyslexia was my dad's insight and knowledge of my love for mechanical objects. He bought an old car motor, against Mom's protests, and informed me that I could tear it apart. He allowed me to use his tools, since I was good about putting them back were I found them. This was the one thing that I could understand easily. I really think my dad was tired of me taking things apart in the house. I would spend hours taking parts off that motor, analyzing what function they had. Each night at the dinner table I would ask dad if I were correct in my assumptions. This went on until my mom, who never mowed the lawn, ran the mower over some parts I had put out in the yard. The mower blade hit an engine part, the part flew out, bounced off the house, hit her in the leg, and caused her leg to turn black and blue. The next day the engine was gone. Mom reminded me daily of how much pain she was in because of me, and I would end up going to my room in tears. For a while I stopped fixing things for her. I did keep a box of "Good Junk" under my bed that I worked on after school. These were items that I had taken out of old toys, clocks, etc., and would make new inventions using them. At the beginning of each week, Mom would throw my good junk in the trash, along with my rock collection. I'd follow behind her picking everything out of the trash.

The ability to take something apart and put it back to its original state gave me self-respect. I could figure out things faster than the neighbor kids. Today, I still have the 1958 Chevy that my dad and brother-in-law gave me to work on when I was 13 years old. The previous owner of the car had hit a cow that belonged to my brother-in-law. According to North Dakota law, if a farmer's cow is hit while it is on the road, the farmer must buy the car. The car was purchased for $300. After sitting for a year, it was given to me. The stipulation was that I had to fix it if I wanted to use it. I worked nights after school, searching for parts, and fixing it up.

My mom also helped with two areas of self-esteem, without even knowing it. One thing she did was give me Legos toys for Christmas one year. That opened many opportunities for me to express myself. I would spend hours working with them. Being dyslexic, I had a talent for seeing a picture of what my creation should look like before even picking up a block. I would outbuild any kid that visited our house. In the fifth grade, I used my Legos to

build a booby trap that shot pencils at my
bedroom door when someone entered . . . that is,
until my mom got hit by flying pencils. It was
soon dismantled, but not until getting each of
my sisters, too.

I soon learned I could out-think other people
in this world and it drove my family up the
wall. One trick was to tape the spray hose open
on the kitchen sink and wait until someone
would go for a drink of water and get, sprayed.
Before I was in sixth grade, I purchased a 101
kit from Radio Shack, and wired the house so I
could listen to what was said in each room and
on the phone. Now that I am older and talking
with other parents of dyslexic children, I have
learned that their children also seem to love
building toys and can make unbelievable
structures with them. This comes from the fact
that a dyslexic child has a strong understanding
of 3-D items.

The second issue of self-esteem my mom
helped with was singing in church. It was hard
for me to read music fast enough to sing along
with everyone in church. In the church song
books, the words were new "shapes" because
they were in segments or pieces for singing
purposes, so I could not read them by
memorization. My mother would help me by
singing the hymns loud, off-key, and a little
ahead of everyone else. I could hear what she

was singing and could then sing along with the congregation by repeating what I had heard. I now live over 1,000 miles from my mom, so I can't go to church and sing next to her every Sunday. This gives me some pain, because at the church I go to now, the minister will stop and ask everyone to sing. I do not sing and do not feel the need to explain why. Sometimes, I just get tired of explaining myself. Church is one place I feel I can go as me, no explanations needed.

I also had trouble learning things that had to be in a particular order. One example is not being able to learn the days of the week or months of the year easily. I would spend hours memorizing the sequence only to end frustrated. Today, in times of high stress, I carry a daily planner in case I have to look up what month comes next.

Another thing that cripples dyslexic children is the SAT test, or any test that requires you to fill the little circles with a number two lead pencil. A dyslexic person will easily lose their place with the line corresponding to the question. Once I finished a timed test with three spaces left to fill and only one more question. On one SAT test, the initial stress of being timed increased my disorientation, causing me to mismatch the answer blanks with the questions on the test. I was unable to correct my answers because time was almost up. SAT should color code each question to match the answer box. I have failed SAT tests because I placed the correct answer in the wrong box. One more reason those tests were difficult was that I read by shapes. For example, in the following test sentence, you are to pick which word is wrong: The buoy ran over to his mom. The word "buoy" should be "boy," but I see it as "buoy." As a dyslexic person I am analytical and can quickly figure out the word should be "boy," because I know that is what is missing in the sentence. On most SAT tests, three words are listed and you are supposed to select the one that is different. Without sentences, I do not understand the words. I might as well stop and flip a coin, because they are out of context. The dyslexic person mixes the sequence of numbers or letters while writing or reading.

Another burden for me as a kid was unmarked water faucets. I have burned my hands more than once. It was difficult to remember which faucet controlled the hot and cold water if they were not marked. It was also difficult to remember that most threaded things, such as screws, were to be turned clockwise for "in" and counter-clockwise for "out." Other simple relationships elude me until I work with them enough that firm patterns develop in my mind. For the most part, these aspects of daily life no longer trouble me unless I am tired, stressed, or have eaten a lot of sugar.

A dyslexic may also have an unusual sensitivity to the contrast of colors. When there is a lot of contrast in colors such as, white writing on a black board, there is a tendency to transpose letters or sentences. I do not know how often I have re-copied a line from losing my place during a class lecture. It was difficult to understand why I could not seem to learn such things while others could do so easily. Someone said it best about this kind of difficulty: "Every difficulty scrambled over will be a ghost to disturb your leisure later on." Even if it was harder for me and took more time, I learned more; not about reading or writing, but reading people, the ways of the world, and knowing when to walk away. Paul Speicher's thought was, " A law of nature rules that energy cannot be destroyed. You change its form from coal to steam, from steam to power in the turbine, but you do not destroy energy. In the same way, another law governs human activity and rules that honest effort cannot be lost, but that some day the proper benefits will be forthcoming." I feel it might not be in the form of your effort, but other strengths will grow.

Chapter 3

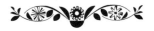

Before looking at other experiences in my life as a dyslexic, I would like to say that my life was not always endless moments of sadness and pain. Not all children tormented me; in fact, some stuck up for me. A special reading group member, Glen, always defended me. He was big for his age and his size scared most kids. We became good friends, and would walk home from school together. His purpose for walking me home was to protect me from the other children, who had grown accustomed to using me as a punching bag. He would defend me from other students and attacks.

This did not go unnoticed, without the other students forming a mob. Glen and I were walking home one night after school, when we saw four or five classmates hiding behind some bushes ahead. We walked slowly, knowing what would happen. They had planned to beat Glen for protecting me. As we got closer, the group of children walked slowly from behind the bushes. They told me to leave, informing me that they would get me the next night. I stayed and watched as Glen was attacked by all five kids at once. They looked like flies hanging on the back of a horse. Glen would turn and hit each kid, giving him a bloody nose or red face. Then each would run off screaming in pain, the same pain they had given me so often. As someone once said, "No good deed goes unpunished."

Their parents called the school, my parents, and Glen's parents. After a long, intense search for the truth, the other kids got in trouble for starting the fight. Glen and I became even closer following this incident. No one bothered us on the way home anymore. My mom told me not to walk home with Glen, even after I explained he was helping me. She felt he was a troublemaker. I am indebted to Glen, and hope to repay him some day.

I have enjoyed many things in my life: working on my car, meeting people who were truly good and not judgmental, learning about the world through dyslexic eyes, and sharing the laughter of my family and friends. God gave me my family, and my family gave me the gift of laughter. Although my family is not always around now, they taught me that laughter is an essential tool for easing life's burdens. I learned that not everyone has the knowledge of laughter, and cannot laugh from the soul. To live life with laughter and love, I believe you must learn it early from your parents.

Another method I use to comfort myself is replaying my fondest childhood memories in my mind. They lift my spirits, filling my head and heart during times of despair. One of these fond childhood memories was the year I went to summer camp. At first I did not want to go because it was a church function, and the top three bullies from school also went to my church. This meant I would have to endure six long days of being verbally and physically tormented. What fun! Sunday school was extra special for these kids, because it gave them one more day of unsupervised privileges. I cried and pleaded with my mom to change churches. Not wanting to burn in hell, we continued going every Sunday. Again, I cried and pleaded. I did everything I could think of, but nothing worked. Mom was still sending me to summer camp for two weeks with my Sunday schoolmates. After arriving at camp, I found that the class bullies had gone to basketball camp instead, so I was safe. The two-week Bible camp had three cabins of boys and three of girls. I was in a cabin with all "special group kids." Our counselor had even attended classes for learning disabilities in his youth. Surprisingly, it ended up being the best two weeks of my life!

There were three highlights from camp that remain in my memory today. First was having the opportunity to compete in camp activities against "normal reading" kids and winning. The second was something my counselor said, "I never knew why God let all those kids do those things to me when I was young. Now I know . . . so I can help you." This came after a night of long talks around a fire, where we each shared our stories and pain of being different. The last and final highlight was winning the prized watermelon at the end of the two weeks by out-thinking the other two cabins.

A contest was held, and the grand prize for having the cleanest cabin for the week was all the watermelon you could eat, and the run of the place for the last night. My cabin wanted to win for all the times we had lost in school because of our reading problems. This victory was to be ours. Unknown to our counselor, we wrote a note and placed it on the door of the leading cabin. The note read, "We do not like watermelon, so do not check our cabin. You can keep it." The other cabin got blamed for the act, because everyone believed we were too dumb to dream up such a stunt. In the end we won by default. After eating the watermelon, we informed our counselor of our trick. He was stunned, but after he paused to catch his thoughts, he burst into laughter.

Throughout these good and bad experiences, I used a measuring rod. I continue to use it today on my current situations. It is based on something Edward G. Bulwer-Lytton said, "Man must be disappointed with the lesser things of life before he can comprehend the full value of the greater."

On the other side of the coin, a haunting memory I used as a measuring staff arrived at the beginning of each school year. As recurring as the yearly flu, winter colds, and shots, it was my personal dark demon that found my hiding place and cast an evil spell on me each year. The immortal spell would change my life and give me a cold slap of reality, which reminded me, "You cannot be normal, Girard. Something is wrong with you." Each year I would begin hoping and praying to God to avoid the unbearable embarrassment and pain. On this day I thought the world had stopped. It was the day I stood out in class and was no longer normal. It was the day I would become

Rudolph the Reindeer after the mud fell off my nose, showing my bright red beacon of dyslexia. This day of terror was the first day of the new school year that I had to read aloud. Those were the days of school I hated most. As Martin H. Fisher said, "Education is the process of driving a set of prejudices down your throat."

Like Rudolph the Reindeer, my social status would change. Now I would be an outcast with the other classmates who were sentenced to the special reading room one hour each day. I would no longer fit in the class, labeled dumb because I could not read without the teacher's help. As if walking over large boulders in oversized shoes, I would stumble over words. Try to picture yourself wearing oversized shoes as you are walking at an incline over large rocks. Now, imagine someone telling you to run fast. As you do, you start falling. Each time you fall, they pull you up, just helping a little, almost as if teasing you. Then they instruct you to run again when you can finally stand. Other children pass by easily, as they say with a laugh, "It's not that hard. What is wrong with you?" For me, this is how it felt reading aloud with dyslexia. I would read as fast as I could, which was slow for the rest of the class. Then I would miss a word. Falling, the teacher would help me just a little, "Sound it out, sound it out." I hated those words as much as I hated, "Let's all take turns reading out of the textbook. Start here and go around the room."

One trick I used was to count the kids ahead of me and try to figure out words that I might have trouble with. I never heard or comprehended what the other kids were reading, so I had no idea what was read while waiting for my turn. As I waited, I would rub my hands together under the desk, water droplets would run down my back, and my heart beat fast. I felt like I had just run as fast as I could on a hot, summer day and then sat. My mouth would grow dry, a lump would form in my windpipe, and I would begin to nervously shake as the child in front of me was reading. I was next in line. The bad thing about being dyslexic is that stress escalates the problem. By the time it was my turn to read, I was lucky if I could read my own name. Speaking softly, I would read the words aloud, missing some, hoping no one could hear. The teacher would always tell me to speak up. I would increase my volume just a little bit and hope the teacher would grow tired of me and move on to the next student. Sometimes this worked and sometimes it had the opposite effect. In either case, once my turn was over, my heart would return to a normal speed and my body would stop sweating. When it came close to my turn again, it would start all over.

The only thing that was worse was when the teacher randomly picked students to read aloud. I would become nervous, not moving, not saying a word, not even laughing when something funny was said. Trying to become a fly on the wall, I felt as if I were in the firing line. It was as if someone was shooting a gun and randomly killing students next to me, and I had no idea if I would be next. The bullet represented the pain of reading, and hearing the children laugh as I missed a word. What died was my self-respect, knowing I was unable to do something that everyone else could.

Reading aloud still creates embarrassment for me today. I avoid it at any cost, especially organizations that require reading aloud (such as Bible study groups or drama clubs). If asked to read aloud, I will stop attending meetings. In the past, I made up excuses with explanations such as, "I do not have my glasses." (I do not wear glasses), or "I have a bad headache, my vision is blurred, and I cannot see the words." Only now do I tell people that I am dyslexic and choose not to read aloud. I found I can only be free if I have the freedom inside to make my own choices. Because of this freedom, I have missed some events I would have loved to attend.

Missing out on school activities because of my dyslexia is nothing new. I would pretend to be sick if I had been beaten up the day before, mentally abused by the teacher and students, or embarrassed by being asked to read aloud. Since I knew how many days I could miss in a given year before being held back, I would pick particular days to miss. Some examples are: when we were required to do an oral reading test, read a report aloud, or, the killer of them all, the day we had the spelling bee test. On spelling bee test day, the class would all stand in front of the room and each person would spell a word until they missed. Well, I always went out fast. It was like I was the largest duck in a shooting gallery and hit first.

As a dyslexic child, these events contributed to my low self-esteem. Imagine that you cannot dunk a basketball. You are instructed to spend eight hours a day trying to dunk the basketball, but with your physical limitations you are unable to. To make matters worse, you are in a group of 30 children who exceed in this skill, but because of the law you must continue spending eight hours a day trying to dunk a basketball. Hopefully, you can now see how this would eventually destroy someone's self-esteem. Would you not do anything to get out of meeting with those people? Would you not play sick, try to be obscure in class, and feel less of a person than everyone else?

This lack of self-esteem soon drifted into another part of my life. What was going to happen when I became interested in dating? I thought it would be like in the movies; I would meet someone, fall in love, and she would understand everything about me and accept me for me. Sadly, I found out that we live in a fast and judgmental society.

As I got older, my folks enjoyed traveling and camping at sites across the Northern states. While camping, I would meet other kids and we would become friends. Now that I had become interested in girls, I would spend more time meeting them. We would have a great time talking, walking along the beaches, taking long hikes, and spending time getting to know each other. Then came the real test of keeping in touch by writing letters after our summer meeting. I would write a letter to my new-found love and go over it, hoping not to make any mistakes. Not letting anyone else check for errors, I would mail the letter. Again, remember my handwriting is also bad. I never heard back from any of the girls I wrote. I am sure if most of you ladies reading this had received a letter from me that looked like a third grader had written it instead of a seventh grader, you would not have responded either. I cannot blame them, but one question stays in my mind—was it me or my writing?

Even if I never wrote to the young women I dated, my dyslexia was still an issue. I would reveal in private that I was dyslexic, and always received the same funny look. Then they would ask if it was hereditary. I was always told I was good looking, but I never believed it because of my low self-esteem. My dyslexia gave girls the perception that I was a slow or dumb person, and this put me on the undatable list. As I sit here typing this on my computer, I wonder if I have become married to my dyslexia, and what would it be like to live without it. This is a question that has always been in my mind and always will. At one time in my life I thought this was all behind me.

My sister Noreen helped me turn my dyslexia into a more positive personality trait. Noreen always reinforced me and told me repeatedly, "You are unique from everybody. Yes, you are going to do stuff differently, but the world needs a variety of people to make it work." This statement and other similar statements helped me . . . especially after Dad moved us to Zap, North Dakota (Yes, there really is a town by this name). After the move, Noreen sat me down and talked to me again. She informed me that I had another chance in a new town, stressing that I should be outgoing, meet people, make a fresh start, and take advantage of the situation. This advice really sank in.

I combined her advice with the help of a future schoolmate, Rick. He had moved from California to Zap the same year I arrived. We met the summer before school started and became good friends. We would spend time discussing our pasts. He could see through my eyes, and helped me with the problems I was trying to overcome. Rick was a true friend because what he advised was not in his best interest, but mine. The biggest gift he gave me was teaching me to enjoy life with friends. He was always there for me, even after I moved away. I could stop in or call him anytime and just talk about anything that was upsetting me. He would always have an answer that made sense. I never got the chance to thank him before he died of leukemia during my senior year.

After Rick's summer help, I was ready for my first day of school, but not for a small town teacher and a class of nine. This meant I could no longer hide in a mass of numbers and fall through the cracks. I was expecting the teachers and the books to be old and outdated. Instead, the books were up-to-date and most of the teachers were fresh out of school. Since I was a first year student, my new principal called me in his office and informed me that I would soon be attending the special reading classes again. I had thought this was behind me and that no one would know about it in Zap. This was to be my new life, my new start. How could this follow me like a bad dream? Little did I know at the time, but a thing called a "file" followed me around. It listed remarks from previous teachers. Fortunately, one thing had changed. I was no longer taken out of the middle of class each day. My special group met while the other eight students had study hall or German class.

Being the only special needs student in a class of nine, I had to meet with students from various other grades. We formed a special secret group. As if a secret oath had been sworn among us, nobody would rat on who was in the group to the rest of the students. Two days out of the week we would meet, hoping that no one would find out. Imagine being with a group each school day and showing your vulnerabilities. You develop a strong bond because of your similarities. Although we did not run around together in high school, the bond was so strong that when I met a member of that special group years later, it was like we still had that common bond and were old friends. There was a comraderie that I have only seen in men who have gone to war together and understand each other better than their own wives, even after having been apart for years.

Since my freshman class only had nine students, I was not able to have one-on-one attention. The disadvantage of going to a smaller school was that some teachers just wanted to get experience and move on. They did not care as much about the students as they did their résumé. These teachers were easy to spot, because they usually did not live in town. If they did live in town, they would leave every weekend for a "bigger" town. One of these teachers was my freshman English teacher. Unfortunately for me, she had no understanding of dyslexia. She thought, as many people still think today, that it is something you outgrow, fix, or my all-time favorite, "He is just lazy." Benjamin Disraeli said, "It is much easier to be critical than to be correct." This teacher informed my parents that I was lazy and just needed to be pushed harder. She said she was going to break me of being lazy. Her justification for my laziness was my sloppy handwriting and my "weird" way of holding a pen. Handwriting for a dyslexic person is anything but neat, and penmanship made up half my grade. Half my points were immediately flushed down the drain in her English class. This teacher must have never read Ralph Waldo Emerson who wrote, "The secret of education lies in respecting the pupil."

Each day this teacher would take time to make fun of my handwriting. She would then throw in a couple of slams about my transposing letters, for which I also lost points. I have to agree with Samuel Johnson who said, "Criticism, as it was first instituted by Aristotle, was meant as a standard of judging well." Evidently she was unfamiliar with Johnson's philosophy, because she was using criticism to punish. She pushed until something snapped. After seeing one of my drawings, a girl in my class said, "I cannot understand why you can draw so good, but you write so sloppy." This hurt, but since I was a freshman, I was not apt to let my feelings show. I looked up to the front of the room and saw my English teacher gleaming with pride. She assumed that since the other students were now placing peer pressure on me, I would snap into shape in no time. This upset me deeply. I was tired of being the object of all her jokes. If I were going to flunk, as she always pointed out, "If your handwriting and spelling do not get better, you'll be repeating this class next year," I was going to go out in style. I snapped all right, and as Dustin Hoffman's character in the movie "Little Big Man" said, "That was the end of my shyness period." My life changed that day and nothing really mattered anymore. After that, I became a walking recording of one-liners from movies and skits I had seen. I quickly gave an answer to that young lady's comment, "I'm just copying pictures when I draw, so why don't you let me copy your homework and I'll have good handwriting?"

My friend Rick was a prankster and had a comeback for each slam, so I guess I was learning this from him. The teacher found no humor in my response, but everyone else did. This was the start of the new me, the clown, the kid who did not really care. If I were going to "crash and burn," then I was going to have fun doing it. I was tired of spending every night trying to do my homework and not getting it right. I was also sick of everyone yelling at me, coming at me with scissors, and people asking me, "What is wrong with you?" After all those years, I had finally discovered a way to let off the steam that had been suppressed. Charlie Chaplin said, "Laughter is the tonic, the relief, the cure for pain."

It took the next year or so for me to fine tune my new found art. Meanwhile, I worked my butt off in that class. Only now am I able to admit to my classmates that the teacher did flunk me in English. I was devastated because it was the first time I had ever flunked a class. Later I found out that she had received a teaching contract from a larger neighboring school system. What a surprise!

My freshman classmates never knew I flunked, because my family moved the next year. This allowed me to repeat English by mail correspondence, and I passed.

When we were planning to move, my parents asked me which town I wanted to live in. I told them I did not want to live in Golden Valley. There had been so many horror stories about that town. If we moved there, I would be one of the few kids who did not wear a cowboy hat. My parents returned from their house hunting trip and informed me that they had bought a house in Golden Valley. So much for my participation in the decision. I screeched with terror at the thought of moving there. To my surprise, it really worked out for the best.

Some of the best times I ever had in school were in Golden Valley, because my classmates were friendly after I settled in. The school principal understood my situation. The special needs classes were held in an old part of the school that no one ever used, which eliminated the embarrassment of being discovered. He also arranged for us to have special education teachers from the county office who were trained well to deal with our problems. My closest friend, who I met at this school, and still keep in touch with today, did not even know at the time that I went to special classes.

Courses like English and history continued to plague me throughout high school. I was a slow reader and those courses always required much reading. Unless I read slowly, the words might look like other words or appear in a "u" shape on the page. I could not keep up with reading assignments, partly because of my slowness, and partly because of my unwillingness to spend much time doing something that did not seem productive. Also, I was still acting as a class clown. To pass tests I would use tricks learned from my past. It worked because I remembered the teacher's comments at conference. My mom came home saying that if I would apply myself to my school work, I could really do well, but then I was just barely passing. In reality, I was working hard while giving the illusion that I was just clowning around.

One trick I used was the association game. Most classes had lectures about what was on the test. As each professor would talk, I would daydream about the item, place, or thing being discussed and illustrate a movie in my mind. At that age I enjoyed picking some well-known lady, who was attractive and sexy. I would imagine the two of us walking down a beach together, and she would softly tell me the things being discussed. Of course, this worked best with the female teachers. I would take notes, but more importantly, I would draw pictures on the side of my note pad that reminded me of the lecture. This is now called mind mapping. I also developed songs and sang them back to the lady on the beach while taking my test. This worked for me, except with the teachers who confiscated my notes because they thought I was just drawing in class. Some teachers gave them back after I explained that I was drawing my notes, but some kept them. I could understand everything when I drew my notes. My life changed for the best. The lesson I learned from this is that life is a game that we all play, and how we play determines how much fun we have. Of course, people still made fun of me, but that was part of the illusion I was creating.

My high school science teacher would tell the class that my handwriting was chicken scratches, and I needed to be neater, but he never really pushed it. Again, most dyslexic students have difficulty mastering the art of good penmanship. I was doing so many other things to draw attention away from my reading and writing that it went unnoticed. Sometimes I would sit in class and dream up stupid questions to ask this teacher. Once I asked him why the sky was blue. He stopped his lecturing, looked at me, and knew he had to answer. This became a game we played in class. Unknown to me, I learned a lot from this game. For the first time I was enjoying school.

My science teacher had a teaching method that worked well for me and helped build my self-respect. Being the drama coach, he also allowed me to have one of the main parts in the school play, which helped my self-confidence. One person can make the difference.

Science became easy, except the written tests, of course. Most of those scientific words are unfamiliar to everyday vocabulary. To overcome this, I dreamed up a new game that put meaning to these words. For example, take the word gluteus maximus. I would take the word gluteus maximums and think, "Okay, my Aunt Gerty (for "gluteus") has a maximum ass for her age." The tests were multiple choice and I could pick out the muscle that was in my aunt's butt. My aunt did not really have a big butt, but it worked.

I really did not stop going to the special classes until I was at the end of my junior year in high school. The principal at Golden Valley tested me by letting me read in class. I could read enough by memorization—and using my tricks— that the principal informed me I no longer needed to continue in the special classes. This was one of the happiest days of my life. I jumped for joy, ran home, and told my mom. It felt as if the world had set me free!

After finishing high school and graduating, I was glad to get out. I knew college was not for me. I did take the ACT test, which only tests how smart you are by how well you can recognize words and fill in boxes. After losing my place on the timed test and filling in the right boxes on the wrong row, I failed badly.

For a dyslexic, taking the ACT test is like viewing a piece of paper with three words on it written in a foreign language. Not doing well on this test reinforced my belief that I could never make it in college. I had been told for the last four years how hard college was, and I was just getting by in high school. I also took aptitude tests and was told I should be an artist or in drama. It seemed that everyone who did poorly on these tests fell into the categories of art or drama. This brings up the question of how many people who take these tests, finish college, and work for years in something they really do not like, just because a test told them to? If these tests truly do work, is it the chicken or the egg theory—the chicken being the personality type in a certain field and the egg being the test directing someone into the field. Which came first? I did contact some colleges about attending their school and most just said my ACT test scores were too low and asked me to retake the test; as if I could do any better the second time around. After all the reinforcing test scores, I thought I could not go to college.

I did not get along with my dad. In fact, we did not talk much unless we got into a fight. He never came to any of my track meets, but had attended my sister Delray's track meets. My father never went to my school conferences although he had attended my sisters'. I really think he was afraid that he was going to hear what my first grade teacher told my mom, and could not bear to hear that his son should be institutionalized. In any heated discussion between my father and me, he would always remind me that I was to be out of the house immediately after my high school graduation. I was still dead to him after all those years.

During my junior year, my folks did not come to a special Parents Day during the basketball season. When the cheerleaders looked for my parents to give them a rose, it quickly became apparent that my parents did not come. I decided then to drop out of basketball. Since my heart was not in it; I was not very good at basketball anyway.

My parents had not saved for my college. I worked nights as a cook to pay for my own clothing, car, car insurance and maintenance, class ring, graduation pictures, graduation gown, etc. I paid for everything except my food and housing. My parents let me live in their home free while I was in high school, but the day after graduation I had to move out. This is what they had done to my sisters, and I was not treated differently.

After graduation, I moved out of the house and into my own apartment. Jumping from job to job, I was looking for my spot in the world. I did about every kind of unskilled manual labor job I was capable of doing, and continued to fill out job applications for good paying jobs with no luck. My handwriting and spelling were holding me back again. I was required to fill out applications in the office and I am sure most of mine fell into trash cans. In the meantime, Noreen kept telling me to go to college. There was a strong notion in my brain telling me I could not go because I would flunk out. I knew what I wanted to achieve, and that was to find a good job that paid well. None of my part-time jobs were going to get me where I wanted to be. So I decided to join the National Guard and did odd jobs for the next couple years, avoiding work that required much reading or writing. But even if the job did not require reading skills the interview required some kind of writing aptitude test. Being dyslexic, I have always failed these tests. I think of these tests as the next generation of the ACT test. Still today, I encounter companies that require some type of testing. I have been tempted to hand in the test blank, with the words, "I'm dyslexic. I flunk," and write "Have a nice day" in Pig Latin. I have lost more jobs due to this type of testing than I care to think about. In 1994 I interviewed with a company that knew my work. An article about me was published in a national trade magazine they had seen. Although I informed them I was dyslexic, they had me take the test anyway. They never called me, avoided my calls, or sent any correspondence telling me I did not get the job. It was as if I had never been there for three interviews. I am glad I did not get the job, because I could not work for unprofessional companies that discriminate against people like me. If they treat me like that after finding out I am dyslexic, how would they treat me as an employee once the interviewing honeymoon was over?

Noreen continued to try to get me to go to college. She realized that I would not get anywhere without it. When I returned from basic training in the National Guard, I decided to try auto body work, because my high school friend was taking a vocational class in it. I found that I could not stand the smell of curing fiberglass, so I spent the quarter just having fun. The general required classes in college were not as bad as the high school teachers had said, at least not in trade school. I believed my high school teachers used college courses as a scare tactic. When we complained about our homework, the teachers would give us details of how hard college courses were. I should have known better. Teachers used the same scare tactics when we were in grade school, only then it was high school classes we were warned about.

I quit school after the first quarter, although I passed English, math, and psychology. I knew I was not destined to make a career in auto body, so I bounced around the countryside looking for something that better suited me. Finally, I ended up in Colorado where Noreen was living. Noreen launched my interest in computers by enrolling both of us in an evening computer class. I went through the class and loved the experience. I was hooked! I could spend all day playing with the computer. It never complained, expected more out of me, or asked anything of me—it just accepted me for me. Noreen borrowed a computer from work so I could have more time to practice, and I got a "C" in the class. Again, I did not do well on the written tests.

I think the teacher liked my sister, since Noreen was attractive and worked well with people. Noreen and I would argue over things in class and he would take her side. One day the teacher stopped the class and asked us how long we had been married and planned to stay married. We both started laughing. The class was quiet and I announced that Noreen was my sister. Everyone said, "Oh," and Noreen began getting even more attention from the teacher. She got an "A" in the class, but she still has to call me for help. From this class, however, I learned that a grade does not always reflect the amount of information one has learned. How you interact with people also has an impact on your grade, and Noreen has great people skills.

I was now hooked on computers, and the invention of the Apple computer was what I had been searching for. I found my field. For one thing, the computer could not yell if something was spelled wrong. I could type the same word wrong repeatedly inside a program and it would be okay. Luckily for me, the computer changed my life. It was very adaptable to my situation, and it would never laugh at me unless I wanted it to.

A computer room always has to be kept at a perfect temperature. It cannot be too hot, cold, or damp. That appealed to me after some of my past jobs, such as working in North Dakota surveying land, up to my waist in water in summer and the wind chill in winter going below zero.

I decided to apply for college in Mayville, North Dakota, and was accepted. Again I packed my bags, and my friends gave me a going away party. I was off to Mayville.

With financial help from the National Guard and student loans, I could attend college, but I was unsure about graduating. Could I get the grades? I had to maintain a "C" average to pass. Although I passed English at the two-year trade school, I feared the four-year college classes would be tougher. As luck would have it, I registered late and all the general requirement classes were filled. So I was able to avoid English for a while, because my advisor really did not care. He was about to move on and was preoccupied with his résumé.

I found out that the role of the advisor is to tell students what classes to take. Not being too respectful of teachers and having had some bad experiences, I decided to pick my own classes, especially after what happened with my advisor. One day I walked into his office. I had only talked to him once before on the phone. After he informed me how much he disliked the new Apple computers, he told me he was one of the original programmers who used copper wires to jump programs together.

My advisor was in his 50's, with gray hair and a small face. He looked like someone who had just lost 200 pounds, and whose suits were too big for him. His hands flew around his desk, scattering the piles of papers as he looked for something. He paused long enough to look at me as I walked in, and yelled as loud as that little man could for me to leave his office. "Get out! Can't you see I'm on the phone?" I looked over to see the receiver lying on the desk next to the phone. So I went out into the hall and filled out my own class schedule by using the book I received from the registrar's office. Then I signed my advisor's name, leaving all my general requirements for my senior year. I never really talked to him again until I had to take a class from him. He kicked me out for wearing a T-shirt that read, "Have a nice day" in big letters, and under it was the word, "asshole." This summed up my attitude.

At this point in my life I really did not care about much. I lived for the moment, having no idea whether or not I was going to finish school. For then, it was something to do. Then something happened that changed my life. I met someone in school whom I cared for and really helped me. A young woman I started dating was taking the same classes as me. We would sit together and, if I had to read aloud, I would ask her about words that confused me.

The classes were small, and I still had to read aloud in class. I could not believe it. My new friend would look over my homework for any grammatical errors also. We dated most of the four years, but it ended. I really never told her how much help she was, and now find myself asking anybody I date to look over things I write. After I explain my dyslexia, as I did to her, I watch how they proof my work. I can read a lot from their reactions, and their sense of caring can be easily detected.

While in college, I got involved in drama, which gave me the self-esteem I needed. I could get up on stage and repeat the lines given to me. And since the lines were someone else's words, I did not have to be accountable for grammatical errors. Another confidence builder was getting involved as a technical director, working with the props, and doing all parts of the show. Being a technical director helped me strengthen my three-dimensional abilities. It really made me feel good when Noreen and some friends from back home would come to my shows. I still love the stage today; It is the only place that feels like home. My experiences in everyday life of playing dumb, sick, and the class clown helped prepare me for the stage. I enjoy community theater, but it often requires cold reading. Since I try to avoid this, I have missed many tryouts. It is hard to act and read simultaneously.

Things were going well for me in college. I was making passing grades, and could pay for the classes and still eat. Besides classes, I was working in the theater and doing drama. I decided it was then time to go for the all-time dream, track. The coach informed me that I was a fast runner, but that was not enough to be on his team, so I was asked to quit track. The truth is, I knew the track coach did not want anybody in drama on his team because these two departments did not get along. It did not take long for the drama teacher to leave under pressure, and the drama department was closed my senior year. Eliza Tabor said, "Disappointment to a noble soul is what cold water is to burning metal; it strengthens, tempers, intensifies, but never destroys it."

This unfortunate experience did not stop me from pursuing my love for drama.

I decided not to pursue my track abilities because my hands were full enough with my new advisor. My original advisor left for a job up north and was replaced with a younger computer professor with a strong background in COBOL computer language. He had worked the mainframe shops and was only exposed to

COBOL, a computer program that uses a large word content and can kill a person with dyslexia. Working with such computer languages not only was unappealing to me, but could also have been disastrous. The possibility of making mistakes or transposing COBOL's long labels and words would have made things difficult for me. My new advisor and computer teacher had little experience in teaching, let alone teaching a dyslexic student. To him, the writing was the most important thing in a program. Unfortunately, I was forced to change my major to business when I began to have problems with the computer classes due to this new advisor.

In the business department, I encountered a professor named Terry. He knew, or guessed, I had dyslexia. In one of my last business classes, he tested us on misused words, which I thought would be a killer. Again, I learned the words by memorization and association. Although it was hard at the time, the way he taught was good and done in a positive way. Terry's teaching style made a world of difference. His classes went by fast because he was full of energy and always started the class out by giving compliments—positive reinforcement to the class or students. He also introduced me to the idea of creating a blue book, which I still have today. I keep copies of cover letters and résumés in it, and I keep updating it with articles that I think are important to me. Terry was a positive influence in my life. I could walk in and talk to him anytime. He was truly a "professional teacher."

I have other people to thank for helping me get through college. Mark, my high school friend, and my sister Noreen (who always knew when to call) showed up for my plays and gave me a sense of caring. I also have to thank God for letting me be creative, so I could get through school. For instance, sometimes I would straighten out a paper clip and use it to make marks on my pen, like a code. I used this to combat the problem of mixing the sequence of terms. For example, in accounting class we had Assets minus Liabilities equals Owner's Equity. My dyslexia would cause me to transpose the order of the words. To remember the order, I would make this mark on my pen " | - | _". This would mean " | " (for one) first letter of the first word and the first letter in the alphabet, "-" stood for minus, and " | _" for "L" in liabilities. I developed other tools. Again, I will use the Assets minus Liabilities equals Owners Equity example. I would take the first letter of each word A - L=O and make a song out of them with the other formulas. The only thing that messed up this system was when a teacher would give multiple choice questions and the answers all started with the same letters. For example: A. Assets - Liabilities = Owners Equity, B. Assets - Liberality = Owners Equity, C. Assets - Libeled = Owners Equity. This was not as cute as the teachers thought, particularly to a dyslexic person who reads by sight. These words were so similar that I could not "see" the differences, making it impossible to choose the right answer. When the test was handed back, the teacher would inform the class that some people picked libeled as an answer.

I find it sad that most teachers have had very little or no training in learning disorders. If they had, they would not have drawn up a test with this question. It would be the same as if you were color-blind and could not see blue, but on a test you were asked to pick out the color blue from brown and black. After taking the first test from a teacher who did this, I became more creative and learned the first and last letters of the word, reducing my chance of error.

I enjoyed classes such as economics, in which my professors educated by using stories to illustrate their point. This made information easier to understand. It was best for me to sit at the front of the room so I was not distracted by other students. I found that smell enhanced my memorization and recall. Different smells remind me of incidents in my past. If I sat beside a young woman who wore the same perfume each day, I did better on tests. I thought about this when I was home and would smell my mom's cooking. If it was something I liked, my mind would jump back to the last time she cooked it for me, creating vivid memories of the time. I knew I could use this to help remember things for my test.

I developed a more controllable alternative in learning. If I sucked on a piece of candy (a different flavor for each class), ate that candy while studying for the test, and again while taking the test, I did better. This helped my memory because I involved more senses in the learning process. Today I can smell something and remember something I learned a long time ago.

None of these techniques worked well when it came to essay questions. My poor writing abilities destroyed me. It would help when the teacher gave us ideas about what the essay questions might be. I could then write out my answers ahead of time and have one of my friends, who was majoring in English, look them over. I would then memorize it as a song. When I hear a new word, especially if it is a new sounding, longer word like dyslexia, it may take me several attempts to pronounce it correctly.

When I was in the play "Oklahoma" I could not get one of my lines, so it ended up going to someone else. Throughout my life, I have tried to ignore and avoid people when they do not accept my disability, as they did in the play. You do not have the time or energy to educate everyone to get them to accept you.

All these incidents were about to end. I was in my final English class of my senior year. We had to write 500 words on a topic we had discussed in class, and we were allowed to work on it ahead of time. After writing it, I had it checked, and memorized the whole thing by putting it on tape and listening to the tape repeatedly as I read along. I did not think I could do it, but I did!

My professors would not remember me for my learning style, but as the student who always wore Army pants. Living on only $115 a month from the National Guard, I could not afford new clothing, especially since I was not getting financial help from anyone. My folks did not approve of me going to school. They voiced their opinion that I should get a real job and stop "playing" in school.

I remember looking at my dad on his death bed, during my junior year in college, waiting for my turn to talk to him. I thought of how he had never even visited me while I was in college; how he had driven around town to visit other relatives but ignored me as if I had some kind of plague. I had offered to pay for everything on parents' weekend, if they would just come down to see me. In return my folks stressed their point by going twice as far in the opposite direction to visit a cousin my dad had verbally wished was his son.

I can still see my dad lying in bed, dying of cancer. He would hold each person's hand and smile at them as they stood beside the bed, until it was my turn. He looked at me with dark brown eyes, which seemed to turn black. The smile dropped from his face and was replaced by his gritting teeth. He yelled for me to get out of his hospital room. It was the day before Father's Day and I had gifts for him. I had just arrived from college after being summoned by my family. I dropped the gifts in a chair and walked out of the room. My sister, who was in the room, cried for me but I could not feel anything. I walked outside where my friend, who had heard the whole ordeal, was waiting for me. We spent all night talking about it and the next day my dad was dead. I had let him down, but how could I do different being dyslexic?

People can change their view of me, but I cannot change being dyslexic. That is why I am writing this book. I hope that teachers and other people will come to understand dyslexia and that one's lack of understanding will allow another child to be hurt.

During my last English class, of my senior year, the college found out I was dyslexic. The college faculty did not wish for me to graduate. There was a big stir at the college because I had this problem and had gotten this far in school. Although I had passing grades, they did not want to let me go into the world with a diploma from their school. The school motto was "The School of Professional Services." After convincing them that I could function in an environment outside the college, and that it was their problem for not catching it ahead of time, they let me graduate. One of my professors had a brother who was dyslexic and she had spotted it right away. Another professor in the same department learned of it and raised a stink. I had been trying to avoid her because I had heard how bad she was. Word about the graduation issue got out and the other students approached me about it.

I was happy to get out of the school with my degree and skin, but I did not leave without receiving some scars from past professors. The college offered a program where I could have three professors write about me and file it with the placement office. The file was never allowed to be seen by the student. After applying for a job I really wanted, a friend at the company informed me I should never use that placement office service again. One teacher did not fill out the paper work at all and another listed things I should not be allowed to do. I should have known better than to use a recommendation from someone who judges writing skills for a living. I was bound to fail. I was only beginning the learning process of real world learning. Wendell Phillips put it foremost, "The best education in the world is that by struggling to get a living."

Chapter 4

After completing the required classes for
graduation, I was physically, mentally, and
emotionally exhausted. This, combined with no
funds for my graduation ceremony expenses
and only Noreen planning on attending, I
decided not to partake in the ceremony.
Instead, I would attend a graduation luncheon
my mother was giving for me at Golden Valley.
Golden Valley was over 300 miles away from my
college. While my classmates were attending
graduation, I packed my white Chevette with
all my worldly belongings and made the last
journey home. I would leave college as I had
arrived, unnoticed, quiet, scared, and unsure of
my future. But now I was wiser. Not so much
book-wiser, but world-wiser.

During my college years I learned some important lessons that would stick with me for the rest of my life. I discovered that in life we often end where we began and see it differently. I was again unsure of the future, but not as scary, because college had been a scary unknown. My high school teachers and elders had drawn a picture of college as a dark demon waiting to eat me alive. They did not think I could ever make it with dyslexia. Being told that some straight 'A' students do not even make it through college did not help. I did make it through college, and learned that people trying to instill fear in me was the only thing to fear.

In reality, college was just a place to buy tools and knowledge for future life needs. That is all it was designed to be. It is not a powerhouse of mad professors playing God with their information. The information is to be used, managed, and understood. The use of learned information in life is more important than any grade I received. Unfortunately, the world judges by the grade and not how the information is applied in life. Since three-dimensional items are my strong point, I can quickly put to work what I have learned, but I am confused at first on the labels or terms. If I were to be tested by a written test, I would score lower than someone who retains terms. If given a hands on test, I would score higher than someone who just retains two-dimensional terms, or better known as "book smart." A writing test is only a test for word retention, not real life.

As I drove into the sunset on my way to Golden Valley, I hoped that the real world would understand my dyslexia more than the college world. In the real world my friends and family had supported me; now it was time to go back and thank them.

At the luncheon in Golden Valley, my relatives and friends congratulated me and wished me luck. After I thanked them for coming and got a good night's sleep, I repacked my car and drove off. I was leaving behind my home, family, friends, and the innocent small town way of life. Down deep I knew I would never return home. I was saying goodbye to North Dakota, childhood friends, and family events. This closed another chapter of my life, and I was leaving all of this to find a new life and a better job market.

The job market in North Dakota was barren for entry level programmers. This is why I had to leave home. One of my college professors told the class we might have to leave the state to get experience before we could come back and get a job in North Dakota. After looking while still in school and discovering that he was right, I decided to look for work in Denver.

I picked Denver because I had met a lady, who I will call Barbara. We had met the summer before and she was now attending school in Denver. We had stayed in touch throughout the school year. Our relationship was good, but unfortunately for her, she would have to experience my problems of being dyslexic and the search for a job.

The job search in Denver was not as easy as I had hoped. It was the summer of 1987 and the job market had gone sour. Denver was overstocked with experienced computer people looking for work. This left few openings for entry level jobs, and the few available entry level jobs in the computer field used two forms of job screening for employee selection. One form, drug screening, was no problem for me; the second was a written test.

Most interviews in Denver followed the same sequence. I would be called for an interview, would arrive on time and then would be seated in a room with other candidates. Each candidate's photo ID was checked and then each was given a test. I would spend the rest of the morning filling in blanks on the test. Upon handing in the completed test, I was thanked for coming, and shown to the door. I was never asked any questions or talked to about the job. Later in the week, I would call only to be informed that I had scored too low to be interviewed.

I failed again because of dyslexia, as was the case with the ACT test in high school. I blundered on the written and reading sections, which lowered my total test score. These low scores were nothing new, which brings up a point I would like to explore. Is the company that fabricates the job screening test the same company that developed the ACT test? Was the company just looking for a new market for their product? If so, it was an easy sell for the salesperson.

I can almost hear the sales pitch for the test to the personnel department,"Simply give the candidate the test, fax it to us, then we will grade it and inform you if the candidate should be hired. You do not have to spend any time interviewing them to see if they can do the job. Just hand them a test and fax it to us. Look how much time we will save you interviewing." Easy sell, but this does not test for any real job skills and only hires one type of person.

This brings up another question on these tests. If a company only hired people who exceeded at two-dimensional tests, do they only employ "A" personality types? If this is true, how can you truly meet the needs of a mixed customer base? Companies that ordinarily use this practice seem to be on the downswing of the business cycle. I have noticed that any new developing field, such as computers, have this life cycle. They grow fast while the creative and hardworking minds are running the fresh company. The field and companies double or triple in growth each year until the companies attract business people which best fit the fields. I like to call these people politicians and documentationers.

The politicians and documentationers have three things in common: they do not get any "productive" work done, they chase out the creative and hardworking people and, they just work on advancing in the company and getting a bigger salary.

The "documentationers" use tons of memos and documentation to flood the hard working group, who are too busy working to protect themselves from the paper war. The "politicians" use golf games or verbal methods to attack the hard working groups who are too busy to play politicians, and soon find themselves out of a job or losing a promotion.

There is a term "business life cycle," that I like to think of as the "business people cycle." People start a company, then someone else comes in to take it over and kills it off. Writing about these people may be just sour grapes on my part, but it was hard not getting past this test and the first stage of the interview. I knew I could do the job, if just given the opportunity. All I was looking for was someone to give me a chance—to interview me or give me a computer and test me on that, not a piece of paper with boxes to fill.

With the tests being used in Denver, no opportunity would come from any of the companies where I applied. While looking for my first break, I worked at a variety of odd jobs. I did everything from delivering furniture to bill collecting to plumbing (my dad always said it was something to fall back on.) As I worked in these miscellaneous jobs, I continued to interview, trying to get a break in the computer field. I was determined to make it, but passing time and growing bills were taking their toll on me. Maybe Denver was not the place for me to look for employment. This would mean leaving Barbara behind.

Barbara was also looking for work, now that she was finished with school. She was having as much unfortunate luck finding a job in her field as I was in mine. She felt Denver was not the place for her to find employment, and decided to return to school in Lawrence, Kansas. Lawrence is a college town, and I knew I could not find work in my field there if Denver was not working out. After hours of talking, we decided it would be best to go our separate ways. It was difficult for both of us, but we agreed it would be for the best. We said goodbye, I returned home to North Dakota, and repacked my car for my next job hunting trip. I had decided to try Phoenix, where a high school friend was working, and I could stay with him until I found something.

Just before leaving for Phoenix, Barbara called and asked if I would stop to see her in Lawrence on my way to Phoenix. While visiting Barbara, I noticed that the Lawrence newspaper was advertising for a Director of Data Processing.

I was underqualified for the job, but I was desperate to find any employment and would apply for any computer position. Not having the required work experience requested in the ad, I remembered what Publilius Cyrus said, "Necessity knows no law except to conquer." So I picked up the phone and called about the job. Dave, who had placed the ad, asked me to stop by his office for an interview. I unpacked my suit, shirt, and tie from my little homeless white car, changed into them, and ran to the interview. The first words out of Dave's mouth, after seeing my résumé were, "Well, that was really gutsy of you, not having the background." He then went on to say, "I'm starting a new company and I need all the software to operate it. Can you write the software to run it?" I told him I could do anything, and that I would do whatever he asked of me. That impressed Dave because that was what he had said on his first job interview. He gave me a hand-held computer unit, a hand-held bar code reader, and told me to take them over the weekend. He said if I could make it do this and this . . . then I was hired. I did what he asked and got the job. Another data processing person, who I will call Bill, was also hired as the Director of Data Processing, and I would report to him.

Bill and I developed systems (accounting, personnel, billing, and general business programs) from scratch. We worked with two PCs and an excellent computer language called C. This was my original introduction to the C language. The C language was well suited for me. It was a pleasure after working with COBOL language in college.

With the language C and the 3-D skills I possessed, I could visualize entire programs and then formulate them in the computer. I had found my true work mate, C and computers, which respected me as I did them.

I had no problem with communication barriers in this environment. The computer forgave my blunders. If I transposed letters, it notified me without screaming—it simply displayed an error message. I was doing good, and enjoyed my work and the benefit of having a steady pay check. Most of all, I was working in my educated field. Again though, all good things must end, or maybe it was God's way of getting me to move on. Either way, things would change.

I worked at this job for over a year with no difficulties, until Bill asked me to submit weekly written reports of my progress week. Because of his request, I revealed to Bill that I was dyslexic, and asked not to do much writing. I tried getting out of doing the reports, knowing that my difficulties with writing would probably blemish me politically. When I submitted my first report, Bill informed me that it, "looked like hell". I was asked to do it over, repeatedly. Bill started to jest and harass me about my writing skills. I found out later this was not the real root of the problem. He could care less about the reports, but he did care about his job and me outperforming him.

Bill was worried about me doing better in programming, and this made him anxious. Since the company was having cash flow problems, he was concerned they would discharge him since I was doing better. Especially since his salary was three times more than mine.

Bill had found something he could use to protect his job, and he could raise himself above me. Our species is made so that those who walk on the well-walked path always throw stones at those who are walking a different path. This was not the only thing Bill could use to protect his job, and throw stones at me.

Something else came up that hurt my standing in the company. Dave, the owner, asked me to generate a letter recalling some bar code units lent to companies. I tried to convince Dave that this job function was best suited for the secretary. Dave did not agree, and reminded me that when I was hired I had promised to do anything. Not having a computer or the money for one, I typed the letter on an old typewriter at home and asked Barbara to proof it.

Barbara was having a bad day, so my request upset her. She stood up quickly from the front room floor where she had been sitting. I can still picture it today: she was in shorts and her hair moved wildly as she yelled and threw her hands around in the air. Her voice was filled with anger and fear—the fear that she had fallen in love with someone who could never hold a good job. This fear was conveyed in the words she said, the words that I will never forget, "How could you get out of school with your problem? Why me? Why do I always have to date the weird ones?" I just stood there and felt a cold rush go through my body as I watched her run out of the room crying.

My first feeling was the pain of someone I loved not understanding. All I wanted out of love was to be understood. I felt the pain of being turned down after getting up the nerve to ask someone I loved for help. It was hard for me to ask for help. It is not easy to show your flaws, especially when so many have laughed in the past. I could not just ask anybody, only someone I hoped would understand my deep secret.

With the pain and hurt of her rejection hanging over me like a black cloud in the apartment, I walked out for some fresh air and away from the sound of her crying. I spent the rest of the night walking around town in the rain. Again, I felt like a second rate human being. That hurt hung on me like a chain around my neck as I walked the streets of Lawrence. The night was misty, foggy, cold, dark, and lonely. Many thoughts went through my mind, but the one I remember the most was something a friend had related to me, "It's better to be alone and by yourself than to be alone with someone." The thought of leaving Barbara hurt more than she had hurt me. We had our share of fights, but I cared too much to get out.

Another thought I had was that maybe I was just dumb and should get an unskilled labor job; maybe I will never make it as a programmer because I am dyslexic. This was reinforced by the voices of kids and teachers from my past. There were many instances to replay in my head that reinforced my low self esteem. It seems that my mind replayed every bad thing that had happened to me, helping me to believe that she was right. I walked around until I was tired and decided to return to the apartment.

When I walked in, I discovered that she had gone to bed, and the letter was untouched. I had thought somehow she would reconsider and work on it while I was gone. Instead, she cried in bed, feeling sorry for herself being stuck with me. This was not the first nor the last time my dyslexia would wound a relationship. As I laid on the sofa, I prayed to God for His help, and that the secretary would understand and help me.

The next morning I painfully asked the secretary if she would proof my letter. I thought it was better to ask her than to let an inauspicious letter go out. She agreed and I handed her the letter, thinking I had found a friend and everything again was okay. I found out later she scanned it quickly and mailed it to over 20 companies. This shocked me, especially since I had helped her with car problems and had given her rides when her car was broken. Yet she did not help me. Unfortunately, the letter contained transposed letters and words. When the letters were received, the phone calls came pouring in from upset recipients. They were upset not only about being asked to return the units, but also with the poor quality of the letter. Companies who received the letters were not the only ones upset.

Dave called me into his office and informed me that, after also being flooded with phone calls, the company that supplied the hardware had instructed him to discharge me. I was flabbergasted that I had squandered my first job, after working so hard and looking for so long. This was not a good week. What was I going to tell my family and friends? What was I going to do? My eyes watered up, my heart hurt, and I felt the same pain as I did a couple of nights before with Barbara. I wanted to escape, but I had no home nearby. North

Dakota was over 900 miles away, with no jobs. I just stood in Dave's office looking at the floor, numbed to the world.

After a moment of silence, Dave saw what I was going through mentally and decided to fire me by "theory" only. I was still employed, but could not use my name for any phone calls or letters. Also, I started doing every garbage job that I once said I would do when hired. I programmed computers, but also painted names in the parking lot, drove people to the airport, picked up boxes from the airport, made name plates, assembled bookcases, and cleaned up messes. This went on for a couple of months, during which home and work stress built up as if the world had been placed on my shoulders. I finally reached my limit and snapped, when physically abused by Bill one afternoon.

I can take the mental and emotional abuse, but physical abuse I do not deal well with. It all came to a head one day when Bill called me an improper name and threw a computer disk across the room, hitting me in the head with it. After being hit, I touched my forehead and felt blood from the computer disk corner hitting my forehead. Bill just laughed and said he was sorry. I cannot remember what else he said, but the blood upset me deeply. The anger grew inside me like fire with gas thrown on it.

Stress that had been bolted down or hidden away inside me was now unleashed and free, rushing through my body, and increasing my anger. The water just started running down my face from my eyes because of the pain and anger inside me. I was crying one of those cries that you do not even know that you are doing. There was no sound, but my body was weeping and my mind was flashing rage. With Bill's treatment of me, I felt I was again being treated like the lowest form of life on earth.

I remember almost falling to the floor as my brain seemed to shut down from the overload of the shock, stress, and anger as each fought for control. Then my brain started again as my temper took the lead. My fist pressed together and the thought of drawing blood from his body, as he had mine, filled my mind. Bill saw the anger in my eyes, halted his laughing, and sat back in his chair, putting his desk between us. I loosened my grip and thought, "No, not that way, I am too proud to do that. This company is not paying me much ($800 a month before taxes.)" I realized it was time to get out and change my situation. Only I could do this. And I would. I walked up to Bill's desk slowly and told him that I made more money doing part-time jobs and that I did not need this shit. Taking my office keys out of my pocket, I placed them in his full coffee cup, and walked out. Since I had my computer programming experience now, more jobs would be open to me. I made the right choice, because I found out the company let most of the other employees go the next year.

As for Bill, he packed his bags one night and left his newborn son and wife, and put a note on Dave's desk saying goodbye. I learned later that he had done this twice before in two other places, two jobs and two other wives and kids. I did learn a lot from Bill before I left, things that a kid living in a small town in North Dakota could never learn. Bill had seen much of the world and different parts of life. He had modeled, acted, and was almost jailed for having drugs and a bomb in the trunk of his car. His stories shocked the hell out of me and caused me to be apprehensive of him and what he could do. To give you an idea of his derangement, he would snicker for hours after feeding his friend's pet snake a chicken for lunch. Bill enjoyed watching how the chicken would try to get away by flying around the cage before getting eaten by the snake. He also told me of a time he pushed a new car down a hill to collect the insurance, because he did not like it after buying it.

With experience this time, I applied for positions while I worked temporary labor jobs. I tried a different approach in my employment search process. Since writing and typing cover letters are not my strong points, I found a secretarial service that could do the job. Every Sunday I would circle the desired position in the newspaper, then Monday morning I would drop by the secretarial service with my ads. The service would develop a cover letter, résumé, and envelope for each ad. It worked well and I was called for several job interviews. I also received more than one job offer within a month. Eventually, I accepted a job with a life insurance company in Kansas City as a PC programmer.

My new supervisor's son was also dyslexic. This was fortunate for me because she could understand my difficulties. She would help me by proofing reports. Ninety percent of my job was programming, so my talents could shine and not be overshadowed by my dyslexia.

My supervisor son's was tested at school and she was told that he was dyslexic. They said her only option for him would be trade schools, something where he could work with his hands. Repeatedly, I tried to explain to her that she should not let anyone set limitations for him.

Too many people have limitations set for them by school teachers, friends, spouse, co-workers, and even themselves. These limitations stops them from doing what they really want to do in life. It is easier to think of a limitation or reason not to do something than to try. The hardest part is to overcome one's thinking. I do not want to sound like one of those self-help tapes going on and on, but maybe reading this will help someone as an article I read helped me. The article was about how someone overcame limitations. It is easier to overcome limitations if you have proof that someone else has done it.

I read an article while working at the life insurance company that changed my life. The article was in a computer mainframe magazine, and the person who wrote the article was also in the data processing field and dyslexic. It became a positive and uplifting event in my life. The author was having the same problems I was, so I realized I was not alone. I hope this book will help someone else in the same way.

When the author of the article was young, he also could not remember which was his left and right arms. I felt relieved, knowing that someone else was having the same experiences. We all form groups and search for people with similarities to be accepted for our differences, and I had found mine.

The person who wrote the article also acknowledged that the computer field was great for someone with dyslexia, because the strengths in it overcompensated for being dyslexic. He preferred to program in Assembler that, like C, worked well for a dyslexic person. Both programming languages have simple short lines of code. He also noted that working with such languages as COBOL, in which a large amount of verbiage was involved, did not appeal to him and could also have been disastrous. The likelihood of mistaking or misinterpreting longer labels and words would have made life hell. He also overcame his inability to read large amounts of material quickly, and learned to shy away from tools or products that would require much reading. In time, he also developed a knack for asking questions and could usually draw a considerable amount of information from the right individual. I found this information joyful. It is my hope that it might also come as a gift to anybody reading this book.

Everything was going great in my job. I loved the work and enjoyed working for my supervisor. This was an answer to my prayers. I could buy new things and could afford to live and feel like I was a part of the human race, not a misfit. At last I thought I had overcome the problems of dyslexia. This too, like childhood, the first job, and everything in life would someday end.

Soon I was haunted by the third ghost of the fill-in-the blank tests. The fill-in-the-blank test company again must have wanted a new market and new way to sell their product. My employer was being haunted and under attack from a hostile takeover. This takeover forced the company to cut costs and people. The data processing department was the biggest area and the first to be cut back.

The screening process would be decided by, you guessed it, a fill-in-the blank test. We were informed in a meeting that each employee would be tested for data processing skills. I could not believe it. I had gotten the job and was doing well. There was even a letter in my file from one of the Vice Presidents on how well I was doing. But I knew the test would somehow erase all of this and put a bad mark in my file.

I was afraid and I could not call in sick. It was mandatory to take the test. If I missed the day of the test, they would reschedule it for me. I was so nervous I had no idea what the questions were or what they were asking. When I finished the test, I knew I had done poorly. At the end of the test, I had one extra box. Somewhere along the way, I had jumped to a different line of answer boxes. Even if I had the right answer, I had placed it in the wrong box. The test came back stamped "this person should not be employed for programming." Fortunately, because I was doing so well in my job, I remained employed. However, this test score would be in my personnel file forever.

No matter how well I did programming, I knew this letter would stop me from being promoted higher than programmer. In my personnel file I was labeled again—damaged goods. After being labeled, I knew I had to move on to another new job with an empty file if I wanted to succeed in my field. Lucky for me, a call came from a company that I had placed a résumé with over a year earlier when looking for work. I was interviewed and hired at Farmland Foods.

At Farmland I worked as a bar coding, automation, and data collection programmer. This was again mostly programming and I could avoid writing reports. Jim, the person I reported to, asked for weekly reports, but did not mind if I made mistakes, accepting them "as is." I also worked with a great group of people that understood my dyslexia. They were open-minded and realized I was talented in other areas, treating me as an equal. My co-workers helped me proofread reports and letters. People really can make a difference.

Each employee was sent to "Seven Habits of Highly Effective People." These Seven Habit classes changed my outlook on life and people.

I understood more about the world and its workings because of this training. The class also started my mind working and thinking higher. For the first time, I truly started breaking down some walls built around me as a child—the walls that kept me in and limited me from doing what I really wanted.

I now had the professional part of my life settled and decided to review my relationship with Barbara. The incident of not helping me with the letter pointed out she had no understanding of my dyslexia; which is more a part of me than the color of my eyes or any other physical attribute. I realized I had a choice and could not live with someone who did not understand my dyslexia. To understand me, you must understand dyslexia and how it affects my everyday life.

There were two options. We could go our separate ways or I could help her understand my dyslexia—and me. I sat with her and tried to explain dyslexia and how it affected me. It was as if she did not want to hear me and again she lost her temper. I did not know how else to get her to understand, so I did one of the hardest things I have ever done by ending our relationship. It is easier if you are on the end of a break up; you have no choice. But if you are the one calling it off, you always wonder if it was the right thing to do. I learned that people can love each other and not live together. With the pain of our break up weighing me down, I knew I had to find a new goal to consume myself, something to keep me busy and drain me by the end of the day. I decided to study for a Masters degree.

A co-worker's cousin was also dyslexic. She received her Masters degree, which impressed me and opened my mind to that possibility. I never even thought I was capable of doing that, so I set it as a goal. Even if a goal is never achieved, at least you tried and learned something along the way.

I called the local colleges with night programs and picked one that best suited me. It would be tough, but I had to try. With a little help from my friends and co-workers, I knew I could do it. Also, I could now afford a computer, which made a big difference in my writing skills. I would use my home computer to write, spell check, and read back my reports. My PC had a sound board, allowing me to do this. It is easier for me to see AND hear the errors than to just see them. After hearing an error, I could fix it.

My PC became my ally and I could find my way around most software without opening a book. I remember sitting in my Masters class with the PC and running through the software without touching a book. The lady sitting next to me was computer illiterate. My PC abilities upset her and she openly expressed her anger in front of the class. She complained that I could move through new software quickly without reading any instructions. Her feelings were that she should be graded differently because she did not understand or work with a PC as I did. Little did she know that this was my survival and I had no choice when she did. The pain of reading the book was more than the pain of finding things on my own.

After finishing my Masters, I thought it was time to move on, so I started applying for other jobs. Soon I was offered a job by another company as manager of automation. I should have never taken this job. During the interview I realized their management style was not one that would understand my dyslexia, but thought I could deal with it. I believed my people skills and work skills were strong enough to overcome their personality types. In the dating arena this is not possible because you cannot change people. I would soon learn this was also true in my professional life as well.

I made the mistake not informing them that I was dyslexic. The company dragged out the interview process for over six months. This should have told me something also. After being hired, I was put into a lower slot than I was offered. The person I was to replace decided not to move into his new position, staying in the one I was offered. I now reported to him, and I will call him Jack. Jack had worked at a larger company and had a knack for writing. He would write somebody to death if he felt he was being "out-memoed." Jack was good at writing and the company we worked for even had him write the corporate report. Jack was a bad manager, changing his mind every five seconds and not caring for those reporting to him. Besides this, Jack did not know anything about automation, computers, or functions of automation, and covered it up by repeating what salespeople told him. He did know how to write and how to play politics. If anybody in the company questioned something he did to upper management, Jack would write many memos and politic them until they were on his side. He loved a good political fight. To give you the last insight to Jack, he first came to the company as a consultant, liked the company, and wanted a job with them. He got his way after playing politics, and was offered a job while in a strip bar after he took his soon-to-be-boss out for dinner and drinks.

Jack felt threatened because I had been working in the automation field for over four years. Also, I got along with the people we did automation work for at the off-site locations. Jack would pick software packages and hardware that the users disliked. Again, this was a power play for Jack, making the off-site location use something they did not want. The off-site location would pick a good product and I would back them in a meeting. This would be the death of my career with this company.

Then Jack found out I was dyslexic. This was the key to getting me out, since he could feel me pushing for his job. He went as far as discriminating against me and teasing me repeatedly about it. In my yearly job review I was chaffed about my communication skills, and told I was unable to do the work because of my dyslexia. Of course, he did not use the word dyslexic, but everything else. Jack also knew that a dyslexia person could not write reports quickly, so that is what he asked me to do. I asked to take them home over night and work on them, but this would not work for him because it would diminish his weapon.

Jack gave me lengthy writing assignments and expected me to have them completed within an hour. I tried to explain to him that, being dyslexic, I needed more time. This only gave him more ammunition and increased his power. Like a mad man hooked on drugs, he wanted more power over me, increasing my work load of nonsense reports. He just kept pushing and pushing. I think he believed confessing my sins lessened his sins. If he had his way, I was going to be the first person that would leave or be fired because of him. Because of software problems with one of his projects, he used other employees as scapegoats. These people were ultimately fired for no good reason. I finally quit, not so much for this, but something else that was revealed to me.

I was traveling on my job entirely too much. At one point, I was out of town for two straight weeks. Jack was keeping me on the road and out of the office, so he could better play his games. The traveling was not what pushed me over the edge. What did it for me was late one Friday afternoon when I walked into the home office after the long two-week trip. I passed one of the owners as I walked up the stairs, carrying a load of books in my arms that I had brought back from an off-site location. The owner was on his way out to play golf. As he met me in the middle of the stairs, he grunted for me to get out of his way. I realized something that day; I was putting up with all this just to make the owner more money so he could play more golf. All my hard work was for someone I did not know or even like. Dawn Steel said upon quitting as president of Columbia Pictures, "You don't resign from these jobs, you escape from them." Also, I was dating a lady at the time that I cared a lot about, but broke up because I was traveling so much. With these two things in mind, I knew what Emile Henry Gauvreaument meant by: "I was part of that strange race of people aptly described as spending their lives doing things they detest to make money they don't want to buy things they don't need to impress people they dislike." I was living a lie, not my life, and unhappy with this lie I was living, so I had to start a new life.

I placed my résumé out in the job market and was very careful with whom I interviewed. Eventually, I took a job as an Information Network Manager at a nonprofit organization, where I still work today. Two people report to me and both know that I am dyslexic. I told the senior director I was dyslexia before he hired me, and found out that someone on the board of directors was also dyslexic. I openly talk about dyslexia at work and know I can never run away from it, but can live with it. Now I can only live with people who accept me for me, what I am, and what I have. I plan to never lower my head to anyone or raise it above anyone.

Chapter 5

This last chapter has been the hardest to finish. It is hard to say goodbye to an old friend after spending so much time with it. I keep rewriting this chapter because of the people I have encountered while developing this book. As I wrote this book, people have asked me what I have been doing with my time. I tell them I am writing a book on my life as a dyslexic person. At first I expressed this in hopes of committing myself to completing the book. Surprisingly, it has become an open forum on dyslexia. It seems everyone knows someone who is dyslexic. This really surprised me, but not as much as some comments and stories I have heard about dyslexic people.

Out of all these comments, there is one that weighs on my heart the most and sticks out in my mind. A man, who I will call Mark, is dyslexic and lived through the same discriminating childhood experiences as me. Because of these experiences, he decided not to have children. In a low voice, so nobody else could hear, he told me he was afraid his children would be dyslexic and have to live through the same hell he did. After hearing this, I tried to help him understand that this disability can have a positive impact to succeed in life. I could not influence his thoughts, because the pain of being a dyslexic child had already been engraved in his mind. My only hope is this book might help him to understand. Dyslexia is something we can overcome, and so can our children, with support and reinforcement from their parents. As Ralph Waldo Emerson pointed out, "Our strength grows out of our weakness." Along with the physical limitations of dyslexia, individuals with dyslexia develop behavioral patterns to compensate for the inconveniences they experience.

Like Mark, I would hide and fear my dyslexia, as a child does with the dark and unknown. It was something I was embarrassed of, and would never tell anyone about it. I have changed, but I am still careful who I tell, not wanting to empower the wrong people. Of course, this will all change when this book is published; then I will have no choice. It is also a waste of my energy and time to explain my dyslexia to someone who just wants "the goods on me" for political reasons. There is a great difference between knowing someone and understanding them; you can know a lot about someone, yet not understand them. I think Mordecai W. Johnson said it best, "When dealing with people, remember you are not dealing with creatures of logic, but with creatures of emotion, creatures bristling with prejudice, and motivated by pride and vanity." It is easier to use the same energy to find somebody who wants to understand and help you reach your goals.

It is important not to let anyone tell you what you cannot do. Decide for yourself what your goals are, and then figure out how to achieve them. Louis D. Brandeis said, "Most of the things worth doing in the world had been declared impossible before they were done." Here is an example: I was told it was impossible for me to write a book. I decided to write a book about my life as a dyslexic person to try to help others. There were a variety of resources to help me with the book: professional services for proofing, transcribing, and editing. One of the major factors in completing this book was the use of computers, along with the support of a good friend to help with the editing. The worst that can happen is this book might fail. As my sister Noreen told me, "If you try and you fail, what's the worst thing that will happen to you? They can't take away your birthday." I decided while writing this book that life is a series of small things in time. What happened yesterday is a small second in your life compared to all the days you will be living. It is best not to let those seconds ruin your days. I would like to say to all people with dyslexia or anyone with a disability—may you overcome it. Franois de La Rochefoucauld said, "Nothing is impossible; there are ways that lead to everything, and if we had sufficient will we should always have sufficient means. It is often merely for an excuse that we say things are impossible."

Another important thing to remember about being dyslexic is your body is a little bit fussier than the average Joe and Jane, so you cannot take your health for granted. Stress can increase dyslexic problems. Most of what I learned about dyslexia has been by word of mouth, such as the following information. Some dyslexic people have a chemical malfunction between the brain and eye. So, anytime chemicals are introduced into the body, the chemicals can increase or decrease the effects of dyslexia. It was explained to me that even the normal eye has blind spots. One example is when you are looking at something in the distance and it is different from it actually is when you get closer. The brain is filling the missing sections with the wrong information. For a dyslexic person, there are more blank spots that the brain needs to fill. This is where the transposing of words and numbers comes in, forcing the dyslexic person to be analytical. I have found that carotene (any green or yellow vegetables) seems to decrease the effects of my dyslexia. These are my theories, not scientific, but things I have noticed. If I eat a lot of fresh vegetables and fruit, the effects are lessened. I have found that some things will affect me such as fruits that have been sprayed. Because of this, I prefer to eat fruits that have an outside skin (bananas, watermelons, or oranges). I can remove any chemical substance that has been sprayed on the outside by removing the skin. This has forced me to become more of a natural foods person. Another thing I have found that has affected me is BHT preservatives, used in everything from deodorant soaps to many breads and cereals. I have actually become allergic to preservatives.

One other piece of advice, for a dyslexic looking for a job, is to be careful. Remember, a company is alive and it has moods and personalities of its own, with each employee being a cell of its body. It is most important to talk to as many people as you can, going into the organization, and finding out if the company's personality matches your personality. If your personality does not fit in with the company, you may be labeled a misfit, overlooked for advancement, and used as the butt of jokes. Remember, in a misfit company there are no victims, only volunteers.

As a child, a dyslexic person is often labeled a slow learner, lazy, or unintelligent. Imagine what kind of low self-esteem a child with dyslexia has. Everyone is an individual and will respond differently to similar situations. In some cases, especially when dyslexia is not diagnosed until later in life, the child may feel alone and inadequate. Other children pick up on peculiarities in each other, and can be quite cruel to others who are different. The dyslexic child's reaction may be to become introverted, turning inward to escape failure and ridicule. Various kinds of avoidance behavior may develop as the young person tries to cope with a world that is hard to understand.

According to the National Department of Health and Welfare, 10-15 percent of school age children in the U.S. are dyslexic, but 75 percent of juvenile delinquents have dyslexia. Could this be from a lack of understanding by both the child and public about dyslexia?

With this in mind, may we learn a little about each other and somehow learn about ourselves or someone we love. I think to understand, we must first begin to communicate, so here is my book to communicate dyslexia to the world. Also remember, as a parent of a dyslexic child, your child needs much attention. Give extra time in learning 2-D figures, along with a large amount unconditional love and encouragement. You need to help your child find his strengths, especially the ability to use 3-D early in life and build on it. Those who have grown up with dyslexia, without being aware of the nature of their dysfunction, need understanding, both of themselves and others. They may need to learn to appreciate themselves so that they look beyond their limitations and exploit their strengths as an adult. Dyslexia is a disability, and to overcome you must do. As Jacques Benigne Bossuet pointed out, "The greatest weakness of all is the great fear of appearing weak."

###

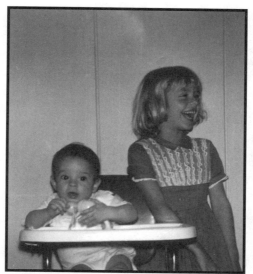

*"At 6 months Noreen was already
looking over me."*

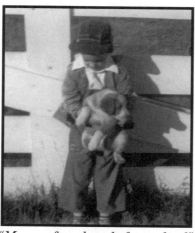

"My carefree days before school"

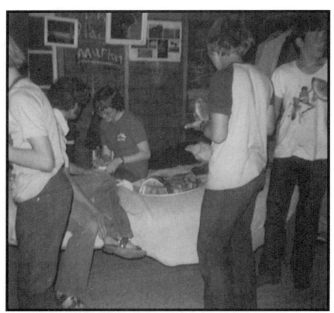

"The sweet taste of victory and watermelon at summer camp."

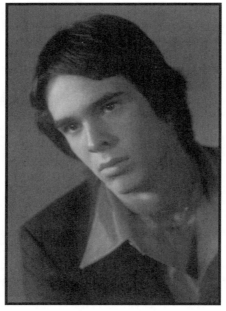

1980 ready to leave behind Dyslexia in high school, so I thought...

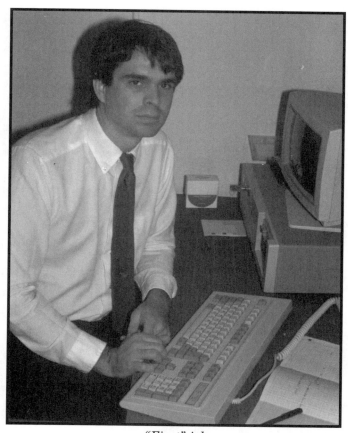

"First" job

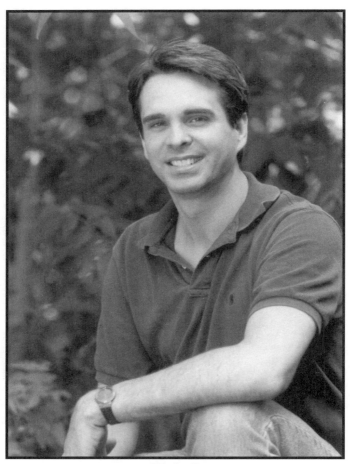

"Today"

Buy additional copies at your local bookstore or use this convenient coupon for ordering. Send check or money order for $8.95 per book - no cash or C.O.D.'s.

Order any quantity you desire.

Send a copy of DYSLEXIA MY LIFE to:

Name:_____

Address:_____

City:_____

State:_____

Zip Code:_____

Send an additional copy of DYSLEXIA MY LIFE to:

Name:_____

Address:_____

City:_____

State:_____

Zip Code:_____

Mail your order, check or money order to:

Dyslexia My Life
P.O. Box 537
Smithville, MO 64089-0537

Any Questions or Comments
Please call 816-803-4679.
Toll Free Visa & MC   (Bookstore)   1-800-428-8309

Thank you for your order...
Email: girards@qni.com
Home page: http://www.qni.com/~girards/

My sister, Noreen's book
Dehydrator Delights
_ _

Visa & MC only   1-800-428-8309

or

Send check or money order

for $7.97 + $2.90 postage and handling.

To: R.R. 1, Box 173
    Moorhead, MN 56560